PREPPER'S
MEDICAL
MANUAL

PREPPER'S MEDICAL MANUAL

THE ULTIMATE READINESS GUIDE FOR MEDICAL EMERGENCIES IN DISASTER SITUATIONS

James C. Jones
Cofounder of Live Free USA

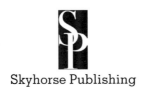

Skyhorse Publishing

Skyhorse Publishing books may be purchased in bulk at special discounts for sales
promotion, corporate gifts, fund-raising, or educational purposes. Special editions can
also be created to specifications. For details, contact the Special Sales Department,
Skyhorse Publishing, 307 West 36th Street, 11th Floor, New York, NY 10018 or
info@skyhorsepublishing.com.

Skyhorse® and Skyhorse Publishing® are registered trademarks of Skyhorse Publishing,
Inc.®, a Delaware corporation.

www.skyhorsepublishing.com.

Cover design by Kai Texel

10 9 8 7 6 5 4 3 2

Library of Congress Cataloging-in-Publication Data is available on file.

ISBN: 978-1-5107-6701-0
Ebook ISBN: 978-1-5107-7489-6

Printed in China

TABLE OF CONTENTS

✝

This book is dedicated to the police, fire, and EMS first responders whose dedication and sacrifice in the face of an epidemic, civil disorder, and chaos is an inspiration to all Americans.

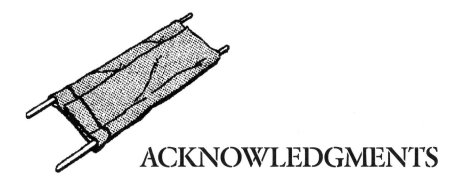

ACKNOWLEDGMENTS

In order to create a thorough and original book, I utilized a wide range of sources and methods. The primary resource was my fifty-plus years of experience as an EMT, survival instructor, industrial safety manager, and first aid instructor. This breadth of knowledge and experience provide a framework to build the chapters on. While I don't claim to know the answers to every first aid question or skill, I did know what questions to address and where to find the answers. In addition to my considerable library of first aid, survival, and medical books, I have notes and memories from dozens of classes and drills. I found that each book covered some subjects well, while over-looking other important issues. EMT training manuals were good at patient evaluation and primary care but assume that the responder will have advanced training and equipment, and immediate access to advanced care. Military manuals focus on combat wounds but do not cover other kinds of medical emergencies. Outdoor first aid books tend to focus on weather-related issues and field accidents. A few texts touched on long-term issues such as resetting dislocated joints or wound closure. Drawing from these diverse sources and my own knowledge, I have tried to create a comprehensive manual for the average citizen who may or may not have access to professional medical help under emergency conditions. In all cases I have made it clear that the first aider should stick to basic "first aid" only, as long as the patient will soon be cared for by professional medical personnel.

Medical aid procedures are difficult to describe without illustrations. Finding or creating effective illustrations and photographs proved extremely challenging. Military manuals are not subject to copyright, and I was able to use illustrations from *Tactical Combat Casualty Care and Wound Treatment*; *FM 21–11, First Aid for Soldiers*, and *FM 21–76 Survival* for some subjects. Having equipment and experience in wound simulation, I was able to create realistic images to illustrate a variety of injuries. These images are simulations; no real blood or tissue was used in their creation. I recruited a few certified first responders to help create images for patient evaluation, CPR/AED, and bandaging and splinting techniques. In many of these, we used improvised material such as torn sheets and pieces of wood rather than premade splints and roll-bandaging. The result was a bit messy but more realistic than overly neat illustrations or professionally modeled photos. In the real world of emergency care rendered by untrained responders, under disaster conditions things will be messy, but all that counts is that it works. With few exceptions, I focused on illustrating techniques that require only one or two responders, as the citizen first aid responder is most likely to be alone or have limited support.

I avoided medical terminology, when possible, As an EMT the term "patient" is the preferable term of those in your care, but I used the more generic term of "victim" when I felt it was appropriate. As this book is intended for the non-professional layman rendering first aid, the term "first aider" is most often used for the person or person rendering care, but "responder" and "caregiver" is also used.

Special thanks to Kimberly Johnson, Trisha Buis, and Marie Jones for helping to create illustrations and photographs for this book.

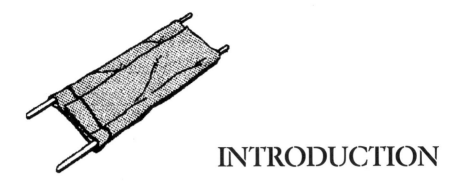

INTRODUCTION

There are dozens of first aid manuals and handbooks on the market, but few are specifically oriented towards the needs of the average citizen faced with a medical emergency under survival and disaster conditions. Military manuals such as *Emergency War Surgery* or *Tactical Combat Casualty Care and Wound Treatment* are intended to be supported by training and available medical support facilities. Basic first aid books like those published by the Red Cross only cover the "first" elements of first aid on the assumption that there will be prompt access to professional medical care. So-called survival first aid books, such as *Ditch Medicine* by Hugh L. Coffee, often focus on field and combat injuries while ignoring more common injuries and ailments. Since the popular image of survival is often associated with outdoor and wilderness situations, there are some excellent texts on those kinds of medical needs including *Wilderness Medicine* by William W. Forgey, MD, and *Being Your Own Wilderness Doctor*, by Dr. E. Russel Kodet and Bradford Angier.

While all of these texts and many more are valuable and provide instructions on how to provide care for various medical situations, they may not meet the needs of the average citizen preparing to meet a broad range of medical emergencies, with limited skills, limited supplies, and limited or non-existent support from the Emergency Management System and medical professionals. I did not want this to be "just another" first aid book. I have approached each subject from the perspective of the untrained citizen trying to provide care for family members and neighbors under extremely trying conditions without help. Of course, I have included all of the basic first aid subjects such as bandaging, splinting, control of bleeding, and treatment of shock, but I have added the following chapters specifically associated with the needs of the would-be prepper responding to true disaster emergencies:

+ Because the survivor may be operating under disaster conditions where there are multiple victims, I have included chapters on triage decision-making, and conscious and unconscious patient evaluation. While professional help may be hours or days away, the information gathered by the initial responders and witnesses may be critical to the victim's recovery.

+ While I have included plenty of information on managing field injuries and environmental illness such as hyperthermia and hypothermia, I realize that most survival situations will occur at home, so I have included chapters on diabetic emergencies, heart attacks, and strokes. These types of emergencies are even more common under the stress of disasters where ambulance response may be delayed or even unavailable.

+ Since this book is specifically intended for those anticipating true disaster survival situations, I have included chapters on scene safety, rescue, victim transport, gunshot wounds, bomb blast effects, communicable diseases, and radiation effects.

+ Being a longtime survivalist and EMT, I realize that the exigencies of providing effective medical care under disaster survival conditions may go beyond basic and legal first aid. I have included some advanced and/or alternative procedures that should be used only when no outside help is expected.

Much of the material in this book is derived from my Survival Medic course and my Eight Critical Medical Skills class as well as my experience and training as an emergency medical technician. I am not a so-called doomsday survivalist living in the wilderness or in a bunker. I was born and raised on the Southside of Chicago and have had periods when I had little access to medical care. As the safety manager of a large industrial facility, I trained and managed an emergency response team and have responded to variety of injuries and medical emergencies. In fact, I was trained as an "industrial medical technician" before EMS classes for first responder and EMT were available.

While first aid knowledge is a critical element in survival, the reader is advised to build a foundation of survival knowledge and provisions. The recent pandemic should demonstrate that dependency on the emergency response systems and life support grid is not a wise course for the responsible citizen of the twenty-first century. Further reading and preparedness is strongly advised. I have written four other books that may be of value to the reader in advancing emergency preparedness and family self-reliance. They are *Advanced Survival, Total Survival, 150 Survival Secrets,* and *The Ultimate Guide to Survival Gear,* all from Skyhorse Publishing.

Handbooks tend to be placed on the shelf or in the pack to be referenced when needed, but I recommend that to be truly prepared the reader should read this book and other related texts to be familiar with the procedures before the need arises. At the very least, be aware of the contents so you know what information is and is not available and can quickly refresh your memory under pressure. If possible, practice the procedures with your family or friends in advance. Such self-training will perfect skills and highlight difficulties. Learning how to render critical care now is far better than learning for the first time under true life or death conditions. Remember that "Emergency preparedness is the duty of every responsible citizen."

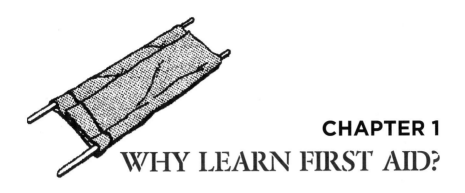

CHAPTER 1
WHY LEARN FIRST AID?

In our system-dependent society where there is an "urgent care" or "fast aid" facility in every community and an ambulance and emergency room within minutes of most homes, first aid knowledge may seem unnecessary. The availability of professional medical help for even minor injuries and conditions has created complacency and helplessness among the general population. Prior to World War II, most cuts, minor burns, strains, sprains, and even some more serious injuries were managed at home.

A good example of this was when I put a nail through my hand as a child. My mother called the doctor, and he said that since I had had my tetanus shot we could just remove the nail and soak my hand in Epsom salt water. In later years I was too poor to afford medical aid. I tore open my knee in a bicycle accident and had to clean the wound and cover it with sterile dressings for weeks while it seeped lymphatic fluids and healed. It left a nasty scar, but that's all. I am sure it would have required stitches and lots of antibiotics, but it healed. I also suffered serious second-degree burns to my hand that were terribly painful for many days. Again, I kept the hand clean and changed sterile dressings, and it healed fine. Historically, there are cases of open abdominal wounds and penetrating chest wounds back when no one knew what to do, but in rare cases the victims recovered.

The recent pandemic and large-scale civil unrest made access to the emergency care facilities and hospitals unfeasible and dangerous. Lack of effective first aid action by family members certainly contributed to many deaths and disabilities that could have been prevented. The social and economic impact of recent events and current trends is likely to result in reductions in the budgets of emergency medical services, as well as fire and police response capabilities, leaving citizens more and more on their own to recognize and manage injuries and medical conditions. The COVID-19 pandemic was not the last major disaster of this century; in fact it has set the stage for a domino effect that will create additional regional and national disasters in the future. While it is difficult to predict exactly what kinds of challenges citizens will face, we can be sure that injuries and illnesses will require the immediate informed actions of family members and neighbors.

All of the preparedness in the world will be of little value if the would-be survivor succumbs to an untreated injury or an unrecognized or untreated illness. First aid must be regarded as a primary survival preparedness skill. The need to acquire first aid skills is founded on practical and moral imperatives.

Practical Imperatives

+ Basic first aid knowledge can be applied to managing everyday injuries and illnesses and help to prevent minor injuries from becoming more serious.
+ First aid skills can be essential when injury or illnesses occur in remote outdoor locations or when professional medical services are unavailable or delayed.
+ In times of local or national disaster, first aid skills and knowledge may be the only thing you have to prevent serious complications, permanent impairments, or death to yourself and those under your care.

Moral Imperatives

+ Being a survivalist or prepper is not a selfish philosophy. By being self-reliant you enable yourself to help others instead of being a burden or a threat to them. The ability to render effective first aid to yourself and others is a civic responsibility.
+ You have the choice of learning to care for and help others, or not learning these skills, but not knowing is not caring.
+ When others are in pain, injured or seriously ill, saying "I don't know what to do" is not morally acceptable. "I don't know what to do" says that you did not care enough about others to learn first aid when you had the opportunity. At that point you are responsible for the suffering and possibly the death of a family member, neighbor, or stranger who needed your help.
+ Being able to render first aid to yourself relieves the community of the need to devote resources to you while it enables you to help others in need.

CHAPTER 2
LEGAL ISSUES WHEN RENDERING FIRST AID

R egardless of the activity one is involved in, the law requires that an individual act or behave towards other persons in a certain and definable manner. Under emergency circumstances the individual will have a duty to act or refrain from acting regardless of training or status. It is expected that the individual will be concerned about the safety and welfare of others when his or her actions may cause injury or harm. The original Hippocratic Oath of "do no further harm" applies. The manner in which a person is expected to act in such situations is referred to as the standard of care. This applies regardless of the individual's level of training. Generally the actions of an individual are judged by comparison to other (hypothetical) persons under similar circumstances with similar levels of training. The person's conduct will be judged taking into consideration the level of training, available equipment, scene safety, and the general confusion and distraction of an emergency. In short: the standard of care is defined as how a reasonable and prudent person with comparable training would be expected to act under similar circumstances, with similar equipment, in the same place.

Under "Good Samaritan" laws those who voluntarily render care to an injured or suddenly ill person are not legally liable for errors or omissions in rendering good faith emergency care. This law applies as long as the actions meet the "standard of care" and "reasonable and prudent person" conditions. Be aware that you may not be immune from responsibility for gross negligence or willful and wanton misconduct. For example: leaving an injured or ill person in cold conditions without providing blankets or failure to move a victim out of a roadway or burning building could be considered negligent; unnecessarily moving a person with a potential spinal injury or trying to administer pills or water to an unconscious patient would probably be considered misconduct.

The first aider should not be administering long-term or advanced medical care for serious injuries or illness when professional care is accessible and available.

While the issues of neglect and abandonment are specific violations for professional first responders they can be applied to the responsibilities of trained and untrained citizens as well. Everyone is expected to do their best to help others regardless of training or professional standards. Ignoring a call for help, failure to call 911 or seek professional care for anyone that you encounter who is injured or ill is a "failure of duty" and can result in both civil and criminal liability. Once you have come to the aid of a seriously ill or injured person you are obligated to provide appropriate care and stay with that person until help arrives. The exceptions to that rule would be if remaining with the person would endanger your life and you cannot safely extricate the victim, or if no further help can be anticipated unless you leave the victim to seek help or call 911.

The exigencies of a true massive disaster with multiple victims, hazardous conditions, and no anticipated medical support will generate challenging situations where doing "the right thing" and doing "the safe thing" may be in conflict. The more you know, the better your decision making will be.

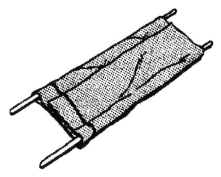

CHAPTER 3
SCENE SAFETY

The importance of scene safety is drilled into every EMT and paramedic and should be a priority for anyone responding to or finding themselves in a medical emergency situation. The principle of scene safety is simple: "Don't rush into an emergency situation and become another victim." Medical professionals have training and protocols to guide them in responding to medical emergencies, but the untrained first aider faced with victims that may be family members or close friends may find it difficult to assess the risks of an accident or disaster scene. Under such high stress conditions, tunnel vision may cause one to focus totally on the patient while ignoring the surrounding conditions. Taking a few breaths while scanning the area and asking yourself, "How did this happen?" and "What hazards are in this scene?" will keep you from being just another victim. Getting yourself injured or killed will not help anyone. Assessing scene safety while evaluating the necessity of rendering medical aid to a seriously injured or ill person is the ultimate risk-versus-benefit decision. In cases where the patient or patients are unresponsive, not breathing, or have obvious arterial (spurting) bleeding, immediate action is required and the benefits of speed may outweigh the risks of entering a hazardous environment, but in most other cases you will have at least a minute or two to gather information from your senses and make a safe plan of action.

Some questions you should ask yourself as you approach the scene or victim are:

+ How did this happen, and are the causes still a threat?
+ What do I see, hear, or smell that could indicate danger?
+ Are there others here that can tell me what happened, or help me respond?
+ Are there others here that may have caused this situation or may be a threat to me and the patient?

✚ Do I have time to make this scene more secure before focusing on rendering first aid?

Some common and often overlooked scene hazards include the following:

✚ Responding to any situation where the patient may have been assaulted, stabbed, clubbed, or shot indicates a high degree of danger to the responder. Do not assume that the assailant or assailants have left the scene or will not return. Carefully examine the surrounding area. Ask witnesses and the patient, if conscious, who caused this injury. Do not assume that witnesses or family members are not the ones who caused the injury or will not assault you as you attempt to render aid. If in doubt, wait for the police or other trusted individuals to provide security while you render first aid. Under true disaster survival conditions, being armed and working with at least one other first aid partner will be extremely helpful.

✚ Any situation where multiple individuals have become ill may indicate carbon monoxide poisoning. The responder can quickly succumb to the same debilitating effects. Get out of the building and get the patient or patients out immediately.

✚ Electrocution hazards are common after a storm, flood, or auto accident involving utility poles and wires. Patient found in flooded basements or anywhere near electrical wires or appliances may be carrying an electrical current. Never enter a flooded or wet area where there may be live wires or charged appliances until the wire has been removed or the power has been disconnected.

✚ Confined spaces such as pits, wells, and tanks can contain deadly vapors or may be oxygen depleted. In some cases, two or three well-meaning rescuers have died trying to help the original victim in such a space. If someone is unconscious in such a space, do not enter. Try to use rope to extricate the victim or try to ventilate the space. Call 911 immediately and let them know that a confined space rescue may be required.

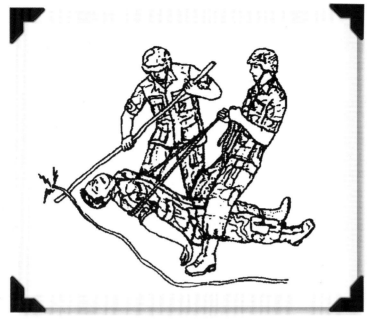

This military manual illustration shows one way to safely remove a victim from contact with an energized wire.

✚ Hazardous chemical vapors or powders can overcome a rescuer if not detected and protected against. Leaking tanks, trucks, or drums may contain ammonia, bromine, insecticides, or other hazardous material. Attempts to rescue exposed victims has often resulted in the death of rescuers. Look for hazard labels. Observe from a distance and upwind if possible. Call 911 and inform them of the hazard and any labels that may be visible.

✚ Storms, earthquakes, and explosions can create unstable structures and dangerous debris. If possible, wait for trained and equipped rescuers to reach patients. If you must attempt a rescue under such conditions wear heavy gloves and head protection. Use available material to shore-up unstable debris and remove sharp debris from your path if possible. Be slow and methodical.

✚ Flammable liquids and gases pose a very serious hazard to the rescuer. If you smell or see gasoline, kerosene, propane, alcohol, or other flammable liquids or gases, be alert for ignition sources. Get yourself and the patient far away from the hazard as fast as possible.

+ Explosions often generate secondary or delayed explosions, gas leaks, toxic materials, and all kinds of sharp fragments. Terrorists often detonate one bomb and then set off another or initiate shooting after the first responders arrive. Be aware of these potential effects and after-effects.

+ Entering a burning building of any kind is extremely hazardous but may be necessary to warn or rescue occupants. Be sure that 911 has been called before entry and be sure others outside know that you have made entry. As the fire progresses, smoke and superheated air will fill the rooms from the ceiling downward, so crawl on hands and knees or crouch as low as you can. Avoid flat crawling because poisonous vapors may result from burning furniture and carpeting.

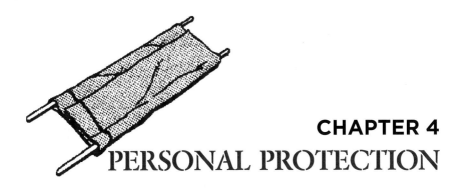

CHAPTER 4
PERSONAL PROTECTION

In addition to making certain that the scene is safe, the first aider may need to protect against contamination from biological hazards. While such concerns may be less urgent when dealing with family members and close associates, strangers may have communicable diseases or be contaminated with hazardous materials that can be transferred to the first aider through contact or inhalation. As part of your scene safety evaluation, you should observe for evidence of contaminating liquids or powders on the patient, and for container labels that may indicate the presence of hazardous contaminants. If there are others present, ask them about the patient's illnesses. In the absence of knowledge to the contrary, assume that the patient may have some form of communicable hazard, and initiate basic self-protective measures. EMTs are trained to don respirators, latex gloves, and eye protection against blood-borne pathogens (BBP) before close contact with a patient.

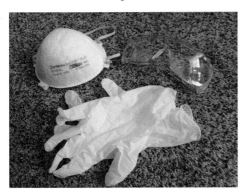

Minimal personal protection includes a dust/mist respirator, glasses or goggles, and latex or vinyl gloves.

Respiratory Protection

Cloth surgical masks are designed to protect the patient against respiratory pathogens from the caregiver, and provide some level of protection against saliva, vomitus, and other bodily fluids. They are not designed to protect against airborne biological or chemical hazards. If the potential for communicable diseases or chemical contaminant is present, properly fitted N95 dust/mist respirators are recommended.

Instructions for Fitting N95 Dust/Mist Masks

1. Mold the nosepiece to the shape of your nose using your fingertips, allowing the headbands to hang below your hand.
2. Press the respirator against your face with the nosepiece on the bridge of your nose.
3. Place the top band high on the back of your head. Move the bottom band over your head and position it below your ears.
4. Using both hands, mold the nosepiece to the shape of your nose.
5. Test the fit. Cup both hands over the respirator and exhale vigorously. If air flows around your nose, tighten the nosepiece. If air leaks around the edges, reposition the bands for better fit.

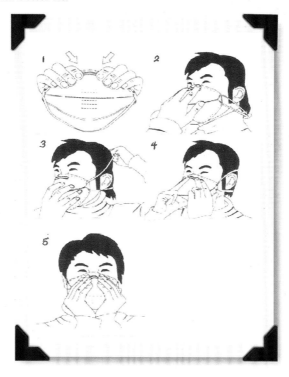

Glove Donning and Removal Procedure

Gloves provide protection for both the first aider and the patient. When putting gloves on, avoid putting your hands on the palm and finger areas of the gloves so as not to contaminate them. Pull the gloves on tight by pulling on the cuffs. Removing the gloves must be done without having your bare fingers contact the potentially contaminated glove outer surfaces. This can be achieved by the following procedure.

Insert the fingers of one gloved hand into the glove of the other hand and pull the glove off by turning it inside out. Slide the ungloved finger of the one hand under the cuff of the remaining glove and pull it downward and inside out. Dispose of the glove into a plastic bag and wash the hands or use hand sanitizer before touching anything.

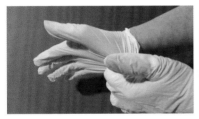

Step one

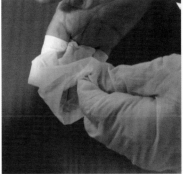

Step two

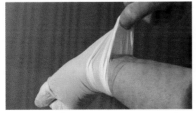

Step three

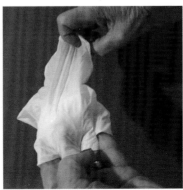

Step four

Eye Protection

Some biological pathogens can be transmitted through contact with eyes. For that reason, eye protection is recommended. Patient actions and the presence of dust and other irritants is also a good reason to have eye protection available. Wraparound glasses are usually adequate to protect against saliva, vomitus, and other bodily fluids, but a face shield is preferable. Fully enclosed chemical goggles are required if toxic or corrosive chemicals may be present.

Protective Clothing

Protective clothing is usually not necessary for first aid situations, unless gross contamination with hazardous substances or infected bodily fluids (blood, vomit, etc.) is present. You can improvise a protective suit from plastic bags, rubber bands, and a pair of surgical gloves. A step better is the basic Tyvek™ chemical protective suits with the hoods and feet. These are cheap (around $12), light, and available in the painting section of most home improvement stores.

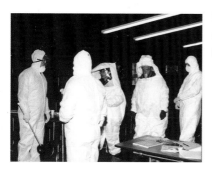

Protective suits are only necessary when dealing with highly contaminated patients.

Decontamination

In cases where gross contamination with biological, or chemical contaminant has occurred, more detailed decontamination steps may be required. Removal of gloves, masks, and contaminated clothing should be done well away from the patient and contaminated area. While complicated decontamination steps are practiced by professional medical and emergency responders, the first aider will be limited to following basic principles:

✚ Do not touch or come close to uncontaminated persons or equipment.

✚ While wearing gloves and respirator, strip contaminated clothing off while avoiding contact with underlying skin and clothing.

✚ Remove the mask with gloved hands avoiding contact with the face.

✚ Remove the gloves following the glove removal procedure.

✚ Wash hands with soap and water or alcohol-based hand sanitizer.

✚ If exposed to aerosol saliva, vomit, or hazardous chemicals, wash the entire body with soap and water giving special attention to the hair, face, hands, and feet.

✚ Contaminated clothing should be disposed of or washed separately.

✚ Equipment exposed to biological hazards should be swabbed or sprayed with a ten percent bleach and water solution.

✚ All contaminated clothing, gloves, respirators, and other items should be placed in plastic bags for safe disposal.

A supply of respirators, gloves, and eye protection should be included in every first aid kit. The potential "Good Samaritan" first aider may want to carry a pair of latex gloves and a flat-fold mask in pocket or purse for unexpected emergencies. Donning these items while doing a scene safety evaluation and triage can provide protection and calm as you begin your initial care.

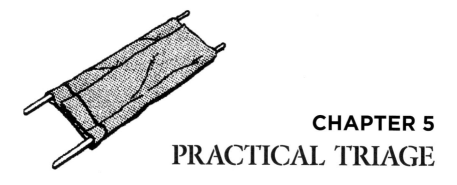

CHAPTER 5
PRACTICAL TRIAGE

Triage is a French word meaning "sorting" and is defined in medical dictionaries as the classification of casualties of war or other disasters, to determine priority of needs and proper place of treatment. Emergency medical personnel use triage to establish who needs immediate treatment, who will require care, and in the gravest extreme who cannot be saved and must be ignored in favor of others. In hospital settings a triage nurse will evaluate incoming patients, sending some to the ER, providing others with first aid, and leaving others to wait for examination in the waiting room. Being effective and accurate at making triage decisions requires a high level of medical training and remains as an educated guess for the professional.

While the first aider may only have to cope with a single injured or ill person, a major disaster could result in multiple victims with a wide range of injuries and only one first aider. Unlike the professional responder, the first aider's triage decisions may be affected by personal issues. Victim "A" may be in more serious condition, but victim "B" may be a close family member or child. Victim "A" may be bleeding to death but may also be the one who caused the injuries to your friends and family. It is unrealistic to expect a civilian first aider to put the lives of strangers or even hostiles ahead of family and friends.

While the responsibility of treating multiple victims can be overwhelming, there are some actions that can mitigate the challenges of the triage process. First: if you can educate your family members in basic first aid skills you will be able to assign them to care for the less seriously injured or even get them started on administration of CPR or application of tourniquets as you continue to evaluate and treat others. You can assign untrained bystanders to hold pressure bandages, get supplies or help in other ways. Those with only minor injuries can even be assigned minor first aid tasks to distract them from their own injuries.

First Look Triage

While detailed examination of each patient will be needed to make a final determination of action priorities, you will be making your first triage decision as you approach the scene. Don't focus on the first victim you see. Examine the scene for other victims while you simultaneously do your scene safety assessment. Since some injuries and conditions (not breathing, severe bleeding) must be treated within seconds of arrival, this first look decision is critical. Victims who are screaming and writhing are conscious and have an airway and therefore can be temporarily ignored, but those who seem to be unconscious may not be breathing and need to be examined immediately. A conscious victim that has spurting arterial bleeding will also require immediate action to stop the bleeding. Your primary survey should be focused on assuring an airway, determination of breathing, determination of blood circulation (pulse), and prevention of arterial bleeding. Cuts, burns, fractures and other injuries can be ignored on the first pass. Always treat life threatening injuries and conditions first, before examining others. Once life threatening injuries are stabilized, you can move on to examination, classification, and caring for less seriously affected victims.

There are several systems for triage, but the system and categories below are the most practical and applicable to scenarios encountered in disaster emergency scenarios. Note that the color codes are those used to tag victims by EMTs and medics in the field or ER. Victims with massive injuries that are obviously fatal are often tagged as black and bypassed but should be rendered comfort when possible.

Category One (Red) applies to victims in need of immediate life-saving action such as airway clearing, CPR, use of an Automatic External Defibrillator (AED), control of severe arterial bleeding, sealing a sucking chest wound, or treatment for shock.

Category Two (Yellow) victims are those who have sustained serious but not immediately life-threatening injuries or are experiencing potentially serious symptoms. Examples of category two situations would include major or multiple fractures, deep or extensive lacerations, extensive burns, chest pain, abdominal pain, head injuries, and those developing hyperthermia or hypothermia. These individuals must be monitored for declining levels of consciousness and signs of shock that may put them into Category One. Category Two victims should receive care and be transported to medical facilities as soon as Category One victims have been stabilized and transported.

Category Three (Green) victims are the "walking wounded" that may have sprains, bruises, abrasions, and other minor injuries that will need medical care or first aid later but can wait or even be recruited to help others.

Category Four (White) are those who will not need any first aid or medical care.

Unfortunately there is an unofficial "Category Five" to be found at disaster scenes. These are curiosity seekers, habitual critics, and even scouts for lawyers. They do nothing to help and often interfere with effective first aid. They may demand to know what you are doing or record your actions on their cellphones. When possible, try to provide the victim with privacy. Say "please clear the area" or "let's give this person some privacy." Certainly if you are in a home, you have the right to ask non-family members to step aside. Be polite, but firmly state that you are doing your best to help the victim and that if anyone has more training they are welcome to help. If a scene safety issue develops, do what is necessary to protect yourself and the victim.

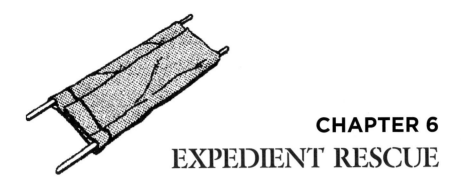

CHAPTER 6
EXPEDIENT RESCUE

In most cases injured or ill patients should not be moved from where they are found since doing so may result in further injuries. Victims of violent trauma such as vehicle accidents, falls, and explosions may have sustained spinal injuries that can result in paralysis if they are moved without effective spinal immobilization. Expedient rescue may be the necessary first priority in rendering first aid under some emergency conditions. While moving an injured person is to be avoided when possible, the location and the environment that the patient is found in may present more danger than the risks involved in extrication and movement. The scene safety observation and mechanism of injuries sustained to the patient may justify expedient extrication on the part of the first aider. Only after the patient is in a safe location can effective evaluation and care be provided.

Justifications for Movement of an Injury Victim

✚ Unstable structures or vehicles where the dangers of further collapse, fire, or movement of debris may endanger the patient and the first aider alike.

✚ Extreme heat, extreme cold, or the presence of heavy smoke or hazardous fumes and gases that endanger the victim and first aider.

✚ Violent environments such as civil disorder, gunfire, and criminal activity is not a safe place to care for an already injured person.

✚ Any location where there is a fire or the danger of a fire such as from spilled flammables or leaking gas must be evacuated immediately.

✚ If the presence of carbon monoxide or other toxic gasses is suspected rapid extrication is justified.

Maintaining spinal stabilization is critical whenever violent trauma is part of the scenario. If the victim is found in an unnatural position and must be turned prior to movement or on-the-spot treatment, the head must be turned gently to the "neutral, eyes front position" that facilitates an open airway and cervical spine alignment. If possible, maintain spinal alignment with gentle traction until a cervical collar can be applied by responders. If this is not practical, use rolled towels or other padded objects placed on either side of the head to maintain the neutral, eyes front position of the head.

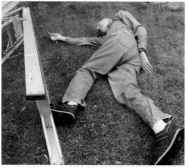

Trauma patients seldom present in good positions. They must be rolled to the prone, eyes front position to assure an open airway, but the cervical spine must be protected and kept in alignment at all times.

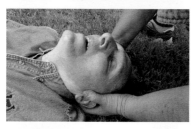

The head is brought to the "neutral" position with gentle traction to maintain spinal alignment.

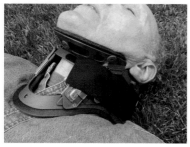

Traction is maintained until a cervical collar or other stabilizing method can be applied.

Basic Drag

If the patient is in a safe location, movement should be avoided, but a basic drag may be necessary if the location is hazardous to the patient or the responder and no one else is available to help. A basic drag can be accomplished by gripping the patient under the arms or on both sides of the shirt collar using the forearms to stabilize the head, while lifting the back and dragging the patient to safety.

Note: Never drag an injured victim by their legs as it may cause severe head and spinal injuries.

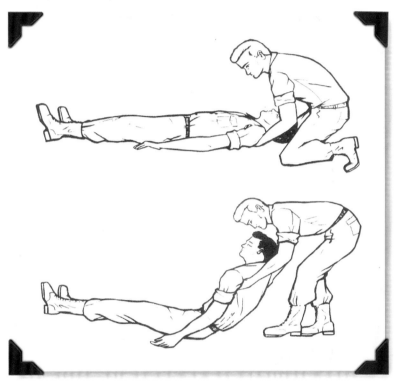

Underarm drag can be accomplished by a single person in an emergency.

Blanket Drag

If a blanket is available, roll the patient onto that and drag the victim to safety.

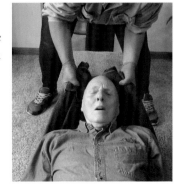

The blanket provides protection, helps to stabilize the spine, and will facilitate transfer to a stretcher.

One-Person or Fireman's Carry

The fireman's carry is an effective way to lift and carry an unconscious patient from a hazardous location. It does require practice and the first aider/rescuer must be healthy and in good physical condition to perform this carry.

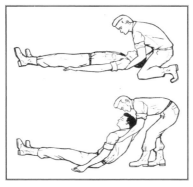

1 Step one is to turn the victim on their chest and reach under their arms.

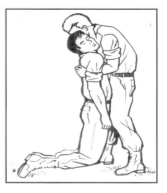

2 Step two is lifting the victim as shown.

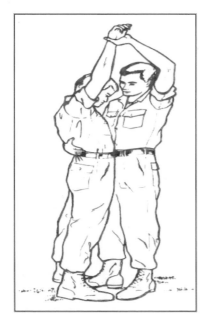

3 Step three is tricky. You must avoid letting the victim fall away from you, or both of you falling backwards.

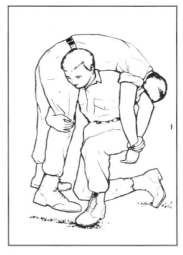

4 Step four is to turn under the victim while kneeling and grasping the victim's arm and leg.

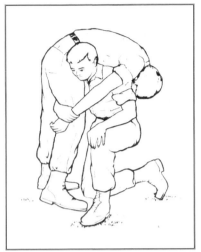 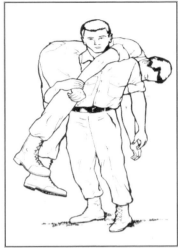

5 Step five is to get the victim over your shoulder while locking the arm and leg as shown.

6 Finally standing and preparing to move. This technique requires strength and practice, but facilitates longer carries.

Two-Person Carries

When other persons are available to assist in a rescue, they should be recruited and instructed to help perform one of the two techniques below. Two-person techniques are faster and safer for both the patient and the rescuers.

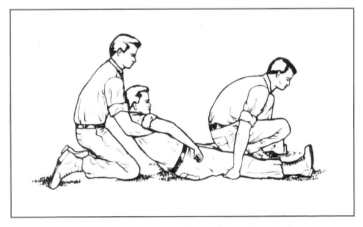

Fast way to lift and extricate a victim for a short distance carry.

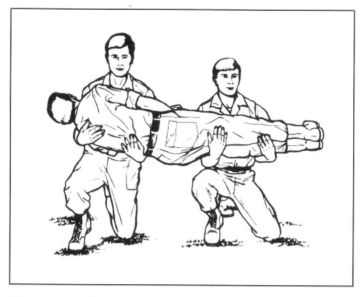

First stage in lifting an unconscious victim prior to carrying.

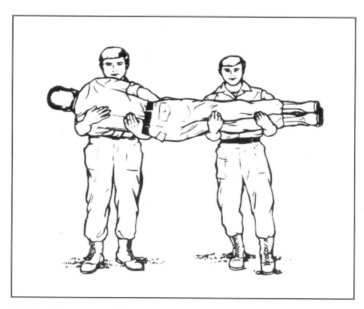

While this method is fast, it cannot be maintained for a long distance, and provides no stabilization for the cervical spine.

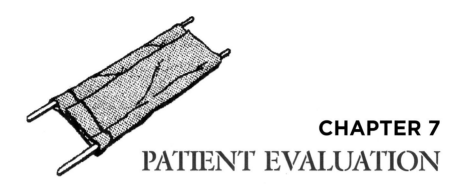

CHAPTER 7
PATIENT EVALUATION

The old medical adage is that there are three important skills to assure effective treatment of the ill or injured patient, "diagnosis, diagnosis, and diagnosis." Failure to recognize or correctly identify the signs and symptoms of a patient's condition can result in delayed or negated treatment, resulting in further complications and even death. First Responders are trained in how to evaluate both conscious and unconscious patients. While the first aider usually just treats the most obvious issues, a more detailed patient evaluation can be valuable under disaster circumstances where access to professional help may be delayed or even unavailable.

Information gathered can help the first aider determine what immediate and long-term actions may be required and will provide information to emergency medical responders upon arrival. With the exception of a thermometer, blood pressure cuff, and stethoscope, the signs and symptoms can be determined using the first aider's own senses. What you hear, see, smell, and feel can provide most of the vital information needed to make informed decisions. Even the patient's temperature and blood pressure can be estimated without instruments. The terms "signs" and "symptoms" are often used incorrectly. Symptoms are things that the patient can tell the responder such as "I have chest pain," or "My arm hurts." Signs are things that the responder observes or determines through examination, such as pulse rate, skin color, limb deformity, or blood pressure.

Primary Survey

The primary survey is directed at establishing that the patient has an open airway, is breathing, and has adequate blood circulation. A conscious patient has all of these attributes and allows the first aider to move on to other diagnostic procedures.

Once it is determined that a patient is not conscious, the first aider must establish that the airway is open. The patient may have choked on something, or the tongue may be interfering with the airway. While kneeling at the patient's side, place one hand on the forehead. Place the fingertips of the other hand under the chin using the thumb to open the mouth while pressing on the forehead to gently lift the jaw and tilt the head. Place the ear close to the mouth to look, listen, and feel for breathing. If no breathing is detected after five seconds, immediately begin CPR. If the patient is breathing, they have at least minimal circulation, and do not need CPR. Severe spurting or arterial bleeding is the other issue with circulation that must be addressed immediately with direct pressure and/or a tourniquet. Once you have a breathing patient who is not bleeding out, you can move on to gathering signs and symptoms.

Level of Consciousness (LOC)

Level of consciousness is the most important vital sign in determination of the seriousness of a patient's condition. Once it is determined that the patient has an airway and is breathing, the patient's level of consciousness can be quickly determined through conversation. The mnemonic "AVPU" can help to remember the levels of consciousness.

+ **A—Alert:** The patient is conversing normally and can answer questions including what their name is, what day it is, and where they are.
+ **V—Verbal:** The patient responds to verbal questions only by mumbling or with unrelated or unintelligible speech
+ **P—Pain:** The patient does not respond to verbal stimulus but reacts to painful stimulus, such as pinching the hand or ear.
+ **U—Unresponsive:** While the patient may be breathing, they do not respond in any way to sound, touch, or pain. This is a very grave sign.

Continuous conversation and observation of all patients is necessary to detect any decline in levels of consciousness over time. This is particularly important for head injuries, significant blood loss, and shock. Any noticeable decline in level of consciousness from the original finding signals the need for early transport and advanced care.

Chief Complaint

The "Chief Complaint" is what the patient tells you about their condition. Unless the injury is obvious, asking an open-ended question such as, "Where does it hurt?" or "Can you tell me what you are feeling?" can provide a guide to your initial actions. Do not ask suggestive questions, such as "Are you having trouble breathing?" or "Do you have chest pain?" that may solicit misleading responses. Do not accept the chief complaint as the only issue. Do a full set of vital signs and patient survey to find all injuries and sources of pain.

Mechanism of Injury

Determination of the mechanism of injury for trauma can be important in assessing the seriousness of an injury and the potential for further complications. For example: A head injury sustained by bumping into a door frame may not be serious, but the same apparent injury sustained in a fall or a vehicle crash could result in a spinal injury or intercranial bleeding. Information that you can provide to professional first responders and doctors may be lifesaving. Important questions could include: How fast was the car going? How long was the knife? How high was the ladder? What did the patient swallow? What caliber was the gun?

Patient's History

While arriving emergency responders will gather this information from a conscious patient, the first aider should try to gather patient's medical history as soon as possible. This information will help the first aider in providing additional care if necessary and can be of great value to medical professionals if the patient later loses consciousness. The mnemonic "AMPLE" is a good guide to gathering this information. This information can be gathered conversationally while determining level of consciousness and conducting you examination.

+ **A—Allergies.** Ask the patient if they are allergic to any medications, latex, or anything they may have eaten or come in contact with.
+ **M—Medications.** Ask the patient what medications they are taking, including prescriptions, over-the-counter, and herbal medication. Ask when they last took their medication. If they have not taken prescribed medication on schedule, they can be aided in taking it if appropriate.

+ **P—Previous Illness.** Ask the patient if they have had any recent hospitalizations or have any ongoing medical conditions.
+ **L—Last food or drink.** Ask when they ate and drank last and what was consumed.
+ **E—Events.** Ask about any events preceding the illness or injury, such as a fall, becoming dizzy, or feeling pain.

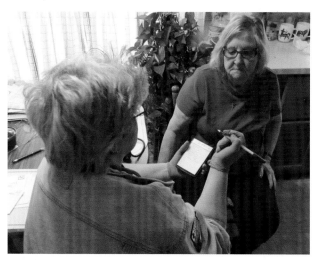

The first step in conscious patient evaluation is determination of the chief complaint, level of consciousness, and medical history. If possible, take notes as the patient may lose consciousness and responding medical personnel will need this information.

Assessing Levels of Pain

The level of pain for a given injury or illness may differ from individual to individual. The fight-or-flight mechanism can generate anesthetics that facilitate temporary pain relief from serious injuries. As with patient history, pain-level assessment can provide valuable help to the first aider and responding medical professionals. There is a big difference between pain from a bump and pain from a potential fracture, and the pain of a heart attack is different from that of a chest muscle strain. The mnemonic for pain assessment is "PQRST" Once the patient has indicated pain or an obviously painful injury is observed, ask these questions.

+ **P—Provoke.** What provokes the pain? This could be movement of a limb, standing up, or any other action that seems to cause or worsen the pain.
+ **Q—Quality.** What does the pain feel like? It may be sharp, crushing, throbbing, burning, dull, etc.
+ **R—Radiating.** Does the pain radiate or move? For example: pain from a heart attack often radiates to the left arm.
+ **S—Severity.** How bad does it hurt? Is it mild, moderate, or severe? You may ask how it compares to the worst pain they have ever had, or on a scale of one-to-ten, how bad is it?
+ **T—Time.** When did it start? Does it come and go? Have you had this type of pain before?

Vital Signs

Establishing the status of vital signs provides information on how the patient's body is maintaining life critical functions. Vital signs that are below established normal levels, or that decline over time, are indications of impending shock or other life-threatening events.

PULSE

The pulse rate indicates how fast the heart is beating. Usually the pulse is taken at the wrist; this is the radial pulse. If the pulse cannot be taken or accessed at the wrist, it can be taken by palpating the carotid artery, just to the front side of the neck. The first aider should count the pulse beats for 15 seconds and then multiply the count by four to establish the rate.

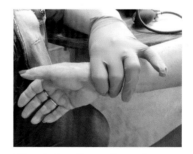

Check for the pulse rate and also the "quality" of the pulse (e.g., bounding, thready, irregular).

Normal pulse rates for adults are between 60 and 80 beats per minute, while children have rates of 80 to 100. A rapid but weak pulse may be an indication of blood loss and shock. An irregular pulse or "skipped beats" usually indicates a significant cardiac dysfunction.

RESPIRATION

The normal adult respiration rate ranges from 12 to 20 breaths per minute Respirations can be counted while taking a pulse. The patient should not be aware that the respiration rate is being taken, as this may make them breath faster or slower. A respiration is one cycle of inhalation and exhalation. Covertly observe and count how many times the patient breathes for 30 seconds then multiply that number by two to establish the respiration rate. Also note the quality of respirations, whether they are deep, shallow, labored, or irregular.

Temperature

The normal oral body temperature is 98.6 degrees Fahrenheit (37 degrees Celsius). In the absence of a thermometer, you can place the back of your hand against the patient's forehead. While this method will not provide an exact temperature, it can provide indications of abnormality. It may feel dry and hot, cold and clammy.

Blood Pressure

Sustaining normal blood pressure is essential to life. Blood pressure below 80 systolic indicates shock and impending death. The systolic pressure (higher number) is established by the heart's contraction, and diastolic (lower number) is the ambient pressure as the heart relaxes.

Normal, adult blood pressure changes with age. The normal systolic reading should be approximately 100 plus the person's age, up to 150 mm Hg. The diastolic (lower number) should be between 65 and 90 mm Hg. Blood pressure may be ascertained using a blood pressure cuff (sphygmomanometer) and stethoscope or one of the many automatic devices. In the absence of equipment, the blood pressure can be estimated based the location of a palpable pulse. If you can feel a radial (wrist) pulse, the patient's systolic blood pressure is at least 80 mm Hg.; if you can feel a pulse at the patient's carotid artery at the side of the neck, the patient's blood pressure is

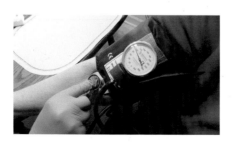

Blood pressure taken with a blood pressure cuff and stethoscope is best, but you can also use an automated wrist device. Blood pressure should be checked about every five minutes to detect any changes.

at least 50 mm Hg. Of course, anything less than 80 mm Hg. is an indication of shock.

How to Take Blood Pressure

The patient must be seated or prone to take an accurate reading. Wrap the cuff securely around the arm about one-inch above the inside of the elbow using the indicator on the cuff. Place the pressure gauge so it is easily visible. Close the valve and pump the bulb to inflate the cuff until a pulse can no longer be felt at the wrist. Place the stethoscope over the brachial artery on the inside of the elbow. Slowly deflate the cuff while listening for a pulse. The gauge reading when you first hear a pulse will be the systolic pressure. Continue to slowly deflate the cuff. The gauge reading when you no longer can detect a pulse through the stethoscope is the diastolic reading.

ADEQUACY OF CIRCULATION

Adequacy of circulation: normal circulation of well-oxygenated blood can be established by pinching the finger tips for a few seconds and then watching for the color to return to the nail beds. This should be "prompt and pink." This is known as "capillary refill."

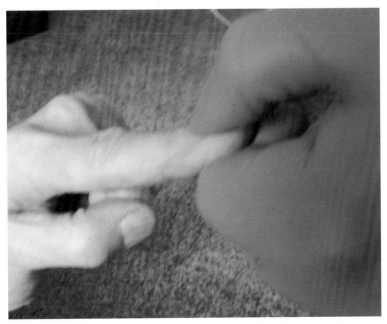

Pinch the finger. The color of the nail bed should return from pale to pink promptly if blood circulation is normal.

ADEQUACY OF HYDRATION

Dehydration results from prolonged illness, heat exposure, and other conditions. Inadequate hydration is an indication and precursor of serious complications. Gently pinch the skin on the back of the patient's hand and watch how it returns to its prior position. Slow recovery indicates poor body hydration.

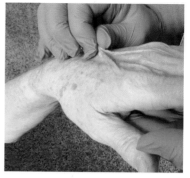

Pinch the skin on the back of the hand; it should recover quickly. If it remains tented the patient may be dehydrated.

SKIN COLOR

Skin color is dependent on the circulation of blood in the vessels of the skin. Changes in normal skin color may be more difficult to detect in patients with deeply pigmented skin, but changes may be apparent in the fingernail beds, on the inside of the mouth, or in the whites (sclera) of the eyes.

Red skin color may be an indication of heat stroke, high fever, or early-stage carbon monoxide poisoning. Later stage carbon monoxide poisoning causes cherry red skin.

Pale, white, ashen skin results from inadequate blood circulation. This is usually associated with shock or cold exposure.

Bluish colored skin, cyanosis, is the result of poorly oxygenated blood. Cyanosis is the result of respiratory insufficiency that may be the result of an obstructed airway or collapsed lung. The cause must be corrected rapidly.

Yellow skin color, known as jaundice, may indicate an illness of the liver or other internal ailments.

PUPIL SIZE AND REACTION

Pupil size and reactivity can be determined on a conscious or unconscious patient. The patient should be out of bright light or should be shaded by the responder. With a small flashlight shine the light in one eye at a time while shading the other. The pupils of the eye should contract quickly. The mnemonic for this is "PEARL," or Pupils Equal and Reactive to Light. Unequal pupil reaction usually indicates a head injury. Constricted pupils in a dark environment

Pupils normal and reactive to light (PERAL)

Uneven dilatation indicative of a head injury

Pinpoint pupils may indicate drug use

Blown (over dilated) pupils indicate deep loss of consciousness or death

may indicate drug usage. Dilated pupils in a bright environment usually indicates unconsciousness or death. Abnormal reaction of the pupil is an indication of central nervous system injury or disease.

ABILITY TO MOVE AND FEEL

When examining a patient who has sustained any kind of fall, impact, fracture, or other violent trauma, the first aider needs to ask the patient to move the injured extremity (e.g., wiggle your fingers. move your foot, etc.) At the same time, pinch the fingers and toes and ask if they can feel that. Loss of the ability to move an extremity or feel pinches may indicate a spinal injury. Immobilize the entire patient with special care to immobilize the neck and head then seek medical help immediately.

Secondary Survey

A full secondary survey, or head-to-toe examination, may not be appropriate for a conscious patient who can provide information on the nature of the illness or injury and direct the first aider to the sources of pain and discomfort. When the patient is unconscious or semiconscious this more detailed examination may be necessary to locate all of the injuries and disabilities. To be effective in locating all injuries it is usually necessary to partially disrobe the patient. The chest, arms, shoulders, legs, and feet must be examined for wounds, deformity, and discoloration, necessitating the removal or cutting-away of clothing. This may not be appropriate for the non-professional first aider. A more focused and discreet examination may be necessary. Examination of the head and face can always be performed.

If possible, this examination should be conducted wearing latex or vinyl gloves.

Head: Palpate the back of the head and scalp feeling for deformities and checking the hand for blood or fluids. Pull the ears forward a bit and check for bruising behind the ears that is an indication of a skull fracture. Look into the ears for fluids or bleeding.

Face: Examine the face for bruising. Examine the eyes for redness or bleeding. Then use a small flashlight to check for pupil reaction. Use the back of the hand to determine the skin temperature, hot and dry, cold and clammy, etc. Observe the skin color. Palpate the facial bones and jaw for deformity. Also note any unusual breath odors that may indicate the presence of alcohol, diabetic ketoacidosis, or other problems.

Neck: Palpate the back of the neck for deformities that may indicate spinal injury. Look for distended neck veins that may indicate cardiac or thoracic problems. Check the position of the trachea. If it is deviated off center this is an indication of a pneumothorax, or collapsed lung.

Note: Throughout palpations of the lower body, continually observe the patient's face for grimacing and listen for sounds that may indicate pain.

Thorax: Observe for equal rise and fall of the chest with respiration. Observe for bruising and penetrating injuries that may also create a sucking chest wound. Gently push on the ribs to detect any fractures. If safe to do so, partially turn the patient so you can observe and palpate the back for additional injuries.

Abdomen: Observe for brushing and penetrating injuries. Palpate for tenderness, rigidity, or pulsing. A firm pulsing abdomen may indicate serious internal bleeding.

Pelvis: Palpate the pelvic area for tenderness. Gently push inward on the outside of the pelvic to detect a fracture.

Legs: Examine each leg for deformity, discoloration, swelling, and wounds. Palpate for tenderness and deformity. Palpate the top of each foot for a dorsalis pulse. If the patient is conscious pinch the toe and ask if they can feel it, then have them push their foot against the resistance of your hand.

Arms: Start by palpating the clavicle and shoulder blade for deformity. Clavicle fractures and shoulder dislocations are very common traumatic injuries. Next examine and palpate each arm for deformity, discoloration, swelling, and wounds. Palpate for tenderness and deformity. Palpate the wrist for a radial pulse. If the patient is conscious, gently pinch the lower arm and ask if they can feel it.

Hands: Have the patient wiggle their fingers and grip your hand to determine strength. This is a good time to pinch a finger to determine capillary refill as an indicator of circulation.

The emergencies of a multi-patient disaster situation may make doing a "textbook" examination difficult, but examination skills and knowing what to look for and how to recognize signs and symptoms quickly is a critical skill for professional and non-professional first aid responders alike.

The head-to-toe survey steps below take about one minute to complete and can identify most injuries.

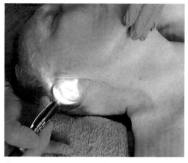

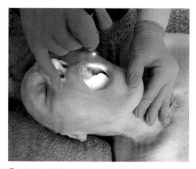

1 Check the patient's ears for leaking blood and spinal fluids. Note the towel-rolls used to maintain spinal alignment.

2 Check the patient's mouth for broken teeth and airway obstructions.

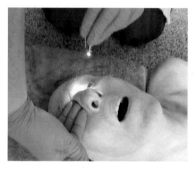

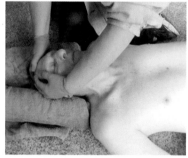

3 Check the patient's eyes for injury and pupil reaction to light. Note covering one eye while checking the other.

4 Check the patient's head, front and back, for deformities and blood.

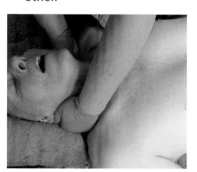

5 Carefully check the neck for deformities and bleeding while minding movement of the cervical spine. While the towel-rolls are temporary spinal immobilization, a cervical collar should be applied as soon as possible.

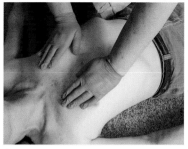

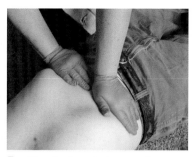

6 Check the chest for broken ribs, sucking chest wounds, and uneven chest movement from a flail chest segment.

7 Check the abdomen for injuries. An overly firm or pulsing abdomen may indicate internal bleeding.

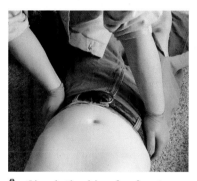

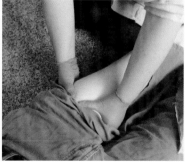

8 Check the hips for fractures by gently pressing and rotating. Listen and feel for grating.

9 Check the thigh and upper leg, front and back, for fractures and wounds. A swollen upper leg may indicate severe, internal bleeding.

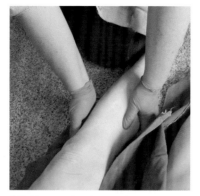

10 Check the lower leg for fractures and wounds.

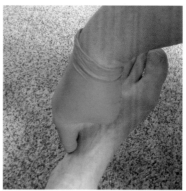

11 Check the foot for injuries, and check the pulse and sensation.

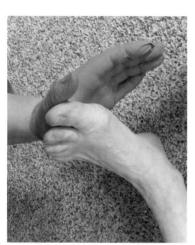

12 Pinch the toe to assess nerve sensation and have the patient push against your hand to assess the ability to move.

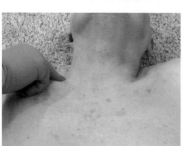

13 Check the clavicle on both sides. This is one of the most frequently fractured bones in the body.

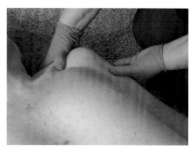

14 Check the shoulder joint for fracture and dislocation.

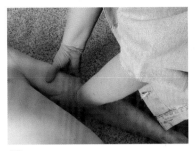

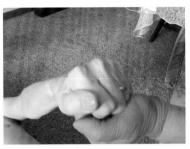

15 Check the upper and lower arm for fractures and wounds.

16 Have the patient squeeze your hand to assess strength.

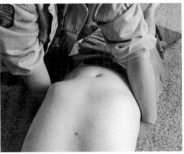

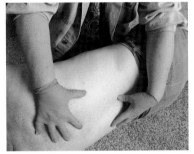

17 While it is best to check the back by turning the patient, this may not be practical if there is danger of a spinal injury. Palpation and frequently checking the hands for blood may be best.

18 Ideally, the patient should be rolled onto their side and a visual and palpation check can be done. If the patient will be placed on stretcher or blanket, they can be rolled back onto that.

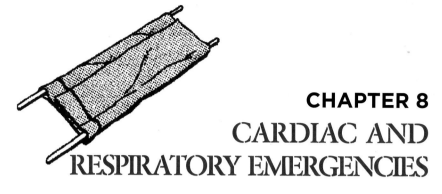

CHAPTER 8
CARDIAC AND RESPIRATORY EMERGENCIES

Assessment

The foundation of basic life support is the maintenance of an open airway, breathing, and blood circulation. These priorities are usually referred to as the "ABCs." Establishing that there is an open airway and that the patient is breathing and has a palpable pulse is the first step in any patient evaluation, and the absence of any one of these critical indicators must be treated before further examination or treatment can be performed.

Obstructed Airway

A sudden airway obstruction in a conscious patient is usually indicated when a person who is eating is suddenly unable to speak or cough. The person with an airway obstruction will grasp the throat, demonstrate an exaggerated effort to breathe and may appear cyanotic (with bluish or purplish skin). Upon observing these signs the first aider should ask, "Are you choking?" If the airway is truly obstructed, the patient will be unable to respond verbally but will nod yes. If the obstruction is not removed quickly, the patient will become unconscious. The following steps must be taken to expel the obstruction:

1. Stand behind the patient with your arms wrapped around the waist. Brace yourself so that if the patient loses consciousness you will be balanced and can lower them to the ground without falling.
2. Grasp one fist in the other hand and place the thumb side of the fist just above the navel, and well below the xiphoid at the bottom of the breastbone.
3. Press your fist with quick strong upward thrusts
4. Repeat this action six to ten times.

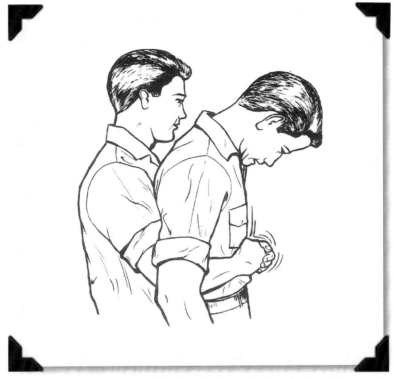

Grasp the patient from behind and place fist just below the navel with the other hand on top. Pull forcefully inward and upward.

This should expel the obstruction. If this fails, the patient will probably lose consciousness.

If a patient is found to be unconscious, first shake them gently and ask "Are you okay?" If there is no response, send someone to call 911, and check to see if the airway is obstructed by tilting the head and lifting the jaw. Look inside the mouth for any foreign objects. Look, listen, and feel for breathing. If no breathing is detected, initiate CPR immediately as for a cardiopulmonary arrest.

If the victim loses consciousness while you are trying to clear the airway, gently lower them to the ground, and send someone to call 911. Examine the mouth for any foreign objects. Look, listen, and feel for breathing. If no breathing is detected, initiate CPR immediately as for cardiopulmonary arrest.

NOTE: Use care in attempting to remove a foreign object from the mouth so as not to push it further in.

Heart Attack (Myocardial Infarction)

The three major possible consequences of a heart attack are sudden death, congestive heart failure, and cardiogenic shock. The objectives of the first aider administering CPR are to prevent sudden death and minimize heart and brain damage. The first priority is to get professional medical services to the patient as soon as possible. While CPR can buy time and give medics a savable patient, it seldom revives the patient without prompt application of an Automatic External Defibrillator (AED) and other aids. Forty percent of heart attack patients never reach a hospital. It is critical that the first aider recognize the first sign of a developing heart attack and call for professional care and transport while the patient is still conscious.

SIGNS AND SYMPTOMS OF A HEART ATTACK INCLUDE THE FOLLOWING:

+ Chest pain described as "squeezing" or "crushing." The patient may say that they "feel like an elephant is on their chest."
+ The pain lasts longer than thirty minutes and is not relieved by resting.
+ The pain often radiates to the left arm, jaw, or back.
+ The patient is not on nitroglycerin for angina.
+ Falling blood pressure as a result of poor cardiac output.
+ Respiration is normal, unless pulmonary edema has occurred causing shallow breathing.
+ Heart attack patients are often extremely agitated and/or experience a feeling of impending doom.
+ The patient's skin will be cold and sweaty and is often ashen or bluish in color.
+ The patient may feel nauseated or even vomit.
+ In severe cases, extended neck veins that do not collapse if the patient sits up may be observed.

MANAGING A CONSCIOUS HEART ATTACK PATIENT

While sending for help is the first priority when encountering a potential heart attack patient, the first aider can take actions to improve the survival chances of the patient while they remain conscious.

+ Reassure the patient and remain calm yourself. While the situation may be serious, alarming the patient will only put further strain on the heart. Talk calmly as you ask about the pain and medical conditions.

✚ Take the patient's history (allergies, medications, previous illnesses, last food and drink, events that preceded the current situation) so you can provide it to responders.

✚ Take vital signs, including: pulse rate, blood pressure, and respiration rate.

✚ Monitor the patient's level of consciousness and alertness.

✚ Position the patient for comfort. This is usually in the sitting position for easier breathing.

✚ If available, send someone to get an Automatic External Defibrillator. No certification is necessary to use one, they are simpler than a cellphone, and they can save a life.

✚ Most importantly: prepare to administer CPR.

ASPIRIN FOR HEART ATTACK

In the early stages of a heart attack, part of the heart muscle is losing its blood supply. Chewing two or three aspirin at this stage can improve the blood circulation to the heart muscle, reducing heart damage or even preventing death. As a first aider, providing two aspirin to someone showing signs and symptoms of a heart attack can make a critical difference in the outcome. Be sure that the person is not allergic to aspirin, and inform medics that the patient has taken aspirin. Anyone older than fifty or who has heart problems should carry aspirin in their pockets and keep them in the bedside drawer.

Cardiopulmonary Resuscitation (CPR)

Various methods of cardiopulmonary resuscitation have been in use for at least one hundred years. The modern version became popular in the 1970s and has been subject to numerous changes since then. The original version was extremely complicated, having different count sequences for every situation. The training required an intense four-hour course, and frequent retraining. Most first aiders forgot which count to use and often froze when faced with an actual cardiac arrest situation. Being afraid to do it wrong resulted in not doing it at all. Recent versions have vastly simplified the CPR procedure and counts so that it can be easily learned and memorized in about one-hour. While official "certification" is desirable, it is not at all necessary. **Anyone who can do CPR should do CPR, without fear of**

legal liability or making errors in technique. The one thing more deadly than poorly performed CPR is no CPR. CPR learned from this book, a video, or a short class will give the otherwise terminal patient a chance to survive. The instructions below are from one of the most current protocols but may not be identical to other past or recent instructions.

✛ Upon finding an unconscious patient, gently shake the patient and shout, "Are you okay?" Be alert for a violent reaction if you have just disturbed a sleeping person. If there is no reaction immediately send someone to call 911 or make the call while continuing your assessment.

✛ Tilt the head and lift the jaw to open the airway. Place your ear next to the patient's mouth. Watch the chest for rise and fall while listening and feeling for air movement for five seconds. (Note that the pulse check in previous versions has been eliminated since lack of respirations will result in cardiac arrest anyway.)

✛ If no breathing is detected, initiate CPR immediately. Place the patient on their back on a hard surface such as a floor, board, or solid ground.

✛ Administer 150 hard and fast chest compressions at the rate of 100 compressions per minute. Each compression should be from 1½ to 2 inches deep. Then check for a pulse. If there is no pulse, resume 30 compressions at the rate of 100 compressions per minute, and then 2 full breaths, until relieved or exhausted.

✛ Alternative: If giving breaths is not practical or appropriate, just administer chest compressions at 100 per minute until relieved or exhausted.

CPR Instructions, Illustrated

Place the patient on their back on a hard surface such as a floor, board, or solid ground.

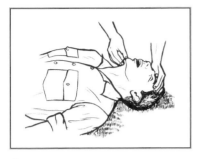

1 Use the head tilt, jaw thrust method to open the patient's airway.

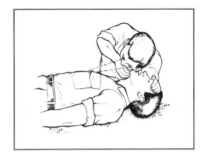

2 For five seconds, watch the chest for rise and fall while listening and feeling for air movement.

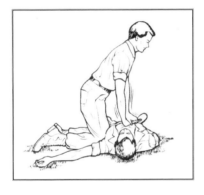

3 Position yourself straight above the patient with the elbows locked, not bent. It is important to use your weight to deliver compressions. Place the heel of one hand directly on the breastbone (sternum) just below the nipple line. Lay the other hand on top of the first hand with the finger interlocked and raised.

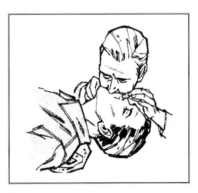

4 Use your body weight to compress the sternum 1½ to 2 inches with each compression. Deliver 30 hard and fast compressions at the rate of 100 compressions per minute. Maintain contact with the patient. Avoid bouncing or rocking motions.

5 Deliver 2 full breaths while placing your mouth over the patient's mouth and pinching the patient's nose closed. Repeat until relieved or exhausted.

Note: Studies have shown that proper CPR with two-inch-deep compressions results in broken ribs in about one-third of patients, but patients who had broken ribs had a higher survival rate due to the effectiveness of the compressions. Don't worry about fracturing ribs.

Automatic External Defibrillators (AED)

While CPR merely sustains circulation, an AED can correct the source of the problem. In most cases the cause of the heart attack is one of two arrhythmias; these are Ventricular Tachycardia (V-Tach) or Ventricular Fibrillation (V-Fib). In both cases, the heart is acting erratically and is unable to adequately pump blood to the brain, vital organs, or extremities. When these arrhythmias are detected by the AED it will deliver a shock to polarize the heart muscle and eliminate the arrhythmias. The heart will then reset and resume normal beating.

Early defibrillators were complex, bulky, and required the skills of trained emergency medical personnel. Seeing these in use may cause the average person to think that using a modern automated defibrillator is beyond their capability. While there are AED certification classes available, and taking one may build confidence, the fact is that anyone can use an AED effectively without training. As with CPR, using an AED without certification poses no legal liability, but not using one when available constitutes a moral failure that may lead to the death of the patient. CPR seldom results in the patient regaining consciousness or recovering without prompt professional intervention, but patients who are afforded defibrillation within the first five minutes after onset of a heart attack have a high rate of survival and recovery. The bottom line is: if there is an AED available, (1) grab it, (2) push the button, and (3) do what it tells you to do. If you can use a cellphone, you are over-qualified to use an AED.

Try not to interrupt CPR. Get someone else to get the AED and have them do CPR or set up the AED.

When you open the AED case, you will see two pads and instructions for where to place them on the patient's chest. It will be necessary to expose the patient's chest to attach these pads. Do not be concerned about propriety, the patient will die if you do not act!

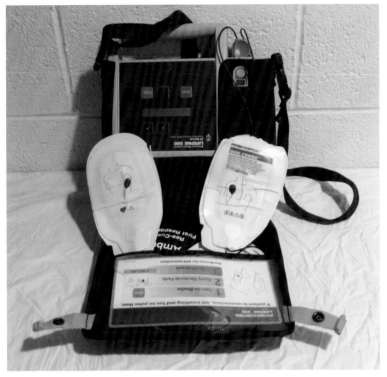

A typical AED. More updated versions have only one button and verbally instruct the user as to what to do next, sometimes with a digital screen display.

USING AN AED

1. Push the activation button.
2. The first instruction you will get is "attach pads."
3. The next instruction will be to "stop CPR."
4. The AED will say "analyzing now."
5. Then it will say "shock advised," or "no shock advised," or "continue CPR."
6. If the AED returns "shock advised," it will usually say "charging now" then "stand clear" followed by "shock delivered" and "analyzing now." With some AED models, you may have to push a button to deliver the shock.
7. Be sure that you are not in contact with the patient when the shock is delivered.

8. After analyzing, the AED will state "shock advised," or "no shock advised," or "continue CPR."

9. If and when the patient recovers consciousness, roll them into the recovery position as they may vomit. Leave the pads in place and continue monitoring the patient.

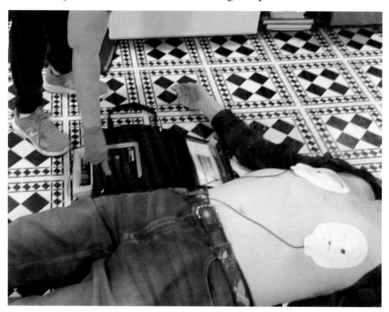

AED in use with pads applied. Be sure that no one is in contact with patient when the shock is administered.

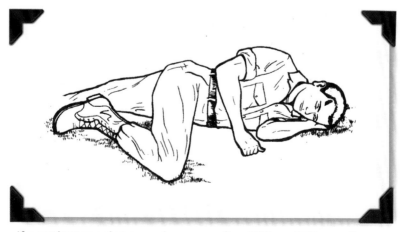

If a patient regains consciousness after CPR or AED use, they should be placed in the "recovery position."

When to Terminate Life Support Efforts

Performing CPR is an exhausting physical activity. One person can only maintain this rate of compressions and breaths for ten or fifteen minutes. If a second or third person is available, let them take over under your supervision. CPR is so simple that even an untrained bystander should be able to do it after watching you. By taking turns you can extend the chances for the patient's survival considerably. You cannot maintain this procedure alone indefinitely if not relieved; your arms will become rubbery and you may even become dizzy. You may not give up, but you will give out.

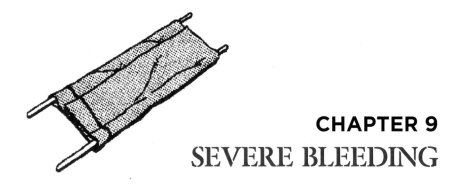

CHAPTER 9
SEVERE BLEEDING

Severe arterial bleeding (hemorrhaging) can result in the death of a patient within one or two minutes unless stopped by the first aider's actions. Venous bleeding is dark red and flows steadily from a wound. This slow bleeding needs to be controlled, but the body can adapt to the loss for a while. Arterial bleeding is distinguishable from venous bleeding by its bright red color and spurting under pressure. The blood spurts out with every beat of the heart at such a rate that the body will be unable to compensate, and hemorrhagic shock and death will occur within minutes. The average adult has about 6 liters of blood. The loss of ten percent (600 ml) or more of this blood volume is very dangerous. Along with airway clearing and CPR, the ability to quickly control arterial bleeding is a primary and essential first aid skill.

The most effective methods of stopping severe external bleeding are the application of direct pressure over the wound site, elevation of the wounded extremity, and application of a tourniquet. While many older first aid manuals listed the application of pressure over arterial pressure points to reduce bleeding, these points were often difficult to locate, and did not fully stop bleeding because bleeding continued through other secondary veins and arteries. Earlier manuals and classes also limited the use of tourniquets to a "last resort" methodology because of the belief that the interruption of blood flow could result in the loss of the limb below the application point. It has been found that tourniquet application seldom results in limb damage if access to professional medical care is available within a short time. However, direct pressure and elevation remain the first step in bleeding control, and a tourniquet should only be used to supplement direct pressure if that method fails to stop the bleeding. Arterial bleeding is a serious medical emergency and 911 should be called immediately upon encountering this type of injury. Surgical intervention and blood transfusion will be required to save this patient.

As soon as spurting, bright red arterial bleeding is observed, the first aider must immediately apply direct pressure over the wound. Use any immediately available piece of cloth or the bare hand as a pressure dressing. There is no time to look for bandaging materials or a first aid kit. Once direct pressure is applied it should not be relaxed. If the blood soaks through the original compress, just pile on more material. Also raise the injured extremity to slow blood flow. Secure the pressure dressing in place with a tight bandage secured with the knot directly over the wound.

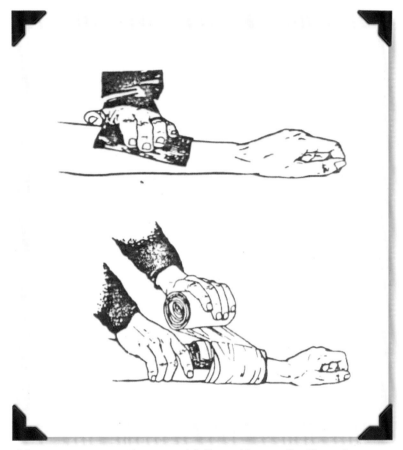

Direct pressure on the wound followed by application of a pressure dressing is usually sufficient to control severe bleeding.

Tourniquets

Direct pressure and elevation are often sufficient to stop even arterial bleeding, but if these steps fail to stop the blood flow, a tourniquet should be applied about two inches above the wound site. While it is desirable to use a purpose-made tourniquet device, a cloth bandana, cravat bandage, or other cloth material can be used.

TOURNIQUET APPLICATION PROCEDURES

1. Fold the bandaging material so that it is approximately three to four inches wide and a few layers thick.
2. Wrap this bandage around the extremity twice a few inches above the wound.
3. Tie a knot in the bandage, place a stick about six inches long on top of the knot, then tie a knot over the stick.
4. Using the stick as a lever, turn it to tighten the tourniquet until the bleeding stops
5. Use another piece of cloth or cordage to secure the stick so that it cannot unwind.

TOURNIQUET APPLICATION PRECAUTIONS

+ Never use wire or narrow material for a tourniquet as it will cut into the skin.
+ Once a tourniquet is applied do not loosen it. This must be done in a hospital where surgical repair and intravenous blood and plasma transfusions are available.
+ Never cover a tourniquet with bandaging, splinting, or clothing. It must be in full view.
+ Always write "TK" and the time that you applied the tourniquet in a piece of tape or directly onto the patient's forehead. This important information for care providers.
+ Never place a tourniquet below the elbow or below the knee. Bleeding in these location seldom requires a tourniquet and application can damage nerves. Direct pressure should be adequate for these locations.

Once the bleeding is controlled, the first aider can proceed to examine for additional injuries, and gather patient information. In all cases where arterial bleeding has occurred, the first aider must anticipate the onset of hemorrhagic shock and commence treatment of that development. Splinting of the injured extremity is recommended to prevent movement and further bleeding.

Tourniquet Alternative: If a blood pressure cuff is immediately available it can be wrapped around the limb above the above the wound and inflated until the bleeding stops. This method is quick and effective but must be monitored to avoid deflation.

TOURNIQUET DEVICES

After tourniquets were reaccepted as a method of bleeding control, a variety of specialized devices came on the market. Tourniquet devices range from the SWAT-T™, which is a simple elastic band, to the CAT™, Combat Application Tourniquet, which incorporates a lever and a locking device. Prices range from ten to thirty dollars. The CAT tourniquets are very effective, but a bit bulky for pocket carry. Police now carry the CAT tourniquet in a belt holster. Small tourniquets like the SWAT-T can be rolled up and kept in the pocket. One of the best all-around tourniquet/bandage devices is the Israeli Battle Dressing. This item can be adapted to almost every trauma situation. The basic dressing/compress is an effective bandage for most wounds, while the elastic bandaging can be used to secure splints or stabilize sprains. The device can also be applied as a tourniquet to stop severe bleeding. The ties are long enough to secure the compress over head wounds, abdominal wounds, and thoracic wounds. Sold for about ten dollars each.

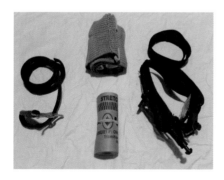

The R.A.T.S.™ tourniquet (left) is fast and effective. The Israeli battle dressing (top center) can be used as a tourniquet, bandage, or to secure a splint. The multi-purpose SWAT-T™ tourniquet (bottom center) is compact and easy to use. The CAT™ tourniquet is the choice of the military and law enforcement.

Application of a Commercially Made Tourniquet to a Severe Bleed

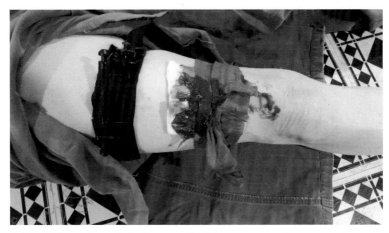

A CAT™ tourniquet device applied to an upper leg wound that already has a pressure bandage in place. Tourniquets are seldom necessary to control bleeding in lower arms or legs.

Application of an Improvised Tourniquet to an Amputation

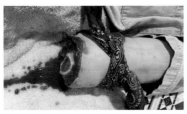 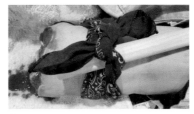

1 A bandana or cravat is tied tightly around the limb about two inches above the bleeding site.

2 A stick of any kind can be used as a lever. Tie a knot over the stick and rotate it until the bleeding stops.

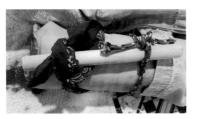

3 Once the bleeding is stopped, secure the end of the stick with any available cordage to prevent it from unwinding.

Blood Stoppers

Hemostatic powders and impregnated gauzes can be used to effectively stop arterial and venous bleeding. Hemostatic dressings are impregnated with a substance that accelerates the clotting process while not sticking to the wound like a normal bandage. If available, hemostatic dressings can be the first pressure dressing applied, but do not delay application of direct pressure to get them. Hemostatic granules can be poured onto an open wound and will stop bleeding effectively. Large hemostatic dressings are especially effective on abdominal and hip injuries where a tourniquet cannot be applied.

The two most established brands for hemostatic agents and dressing are Celox™, and QuikClot®. Z-fold hemostatic gauzes are long strips of narrow (usually one-inch wide) impregnated material that can be stuffed into an open wound to stop bleeding. Celox makes an application plunger device that is inserted into a deep puncture wound such as a gunshot wound, then the plunger is pushed to inject hemostatic granules that will seal the wound. Hemostatic powders can be poured onto or into any open wound.

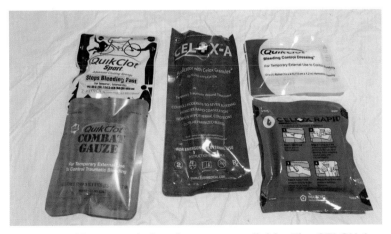

A variety of hemostatic bandages are available. The CELOX-A (center) is an injector of hemostatic particles specifically for use on gunshot wounds.

Internal Bleeding

Profuse and arterial bleeding may occur from violent trauma, without external wounds. Major blood vessels may be ruptured, hemorrhaging blood into body tissues, organs, and cavities. Internal bleeding into an extremity may be indicated by massive bruising and swelling, accompanied by signs and symptoms of shock. Application of splints and tight bandaging may help to reduce internal bleeding, but tourniquets are generally not effective or recommended. The patient must be transported to professional medical facilities immediately to prevent serious or fatal consequences.

While the first aider cannot do much the control internal bleeding into the abdomen or thorax, it is important to be able to recognize the signs. These include:

✚ Vomiting, or coughing up of bright red blood
✚ Black tar-like stools
✚ Bleeding from the rectum
✚ Blood in the urine
✚ Black or blue discoloration of the skin (Ecchymosis)
✚ A mass of blood accumulated beneath the skin, known as a hematoma

Any of these signs is evident of a serious medical problem that requires prompt professional attention. Treat any patient with internal bleeding for shock and anticipate vomiting. Control any sources of external bleeding and splint injured limbs. Keep the patient calm and immobile, as movement may exacerbate bleeding.

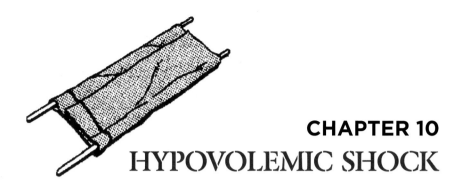

CHAPTER 10
HYPOVOLEMIC SHOCK

Hypovolemic shock, also known as hemorrhagic shock, usually results from significant blood loss due to severe external or internal bleeding. Low blood volume and hypovolemic shock can also develop as a result of severe thermal burns where plasma leaks from the circulatory system into the burned tissue. If the patient is dehydrated prior to injury, shock may develop more rapidly from bleeding. When blood volume drops, circulation becomes inadequate to supply the vital organs and shock develops. Shock should be expected to develop in all cases of severe bleeding or violent trauma.

The following are the most common signs and symptoms of shock:

1. Restlessness and anxiety are often the first signs of impending shock.
2. A weak and rapid pulse that may be difficult to feel.
3. Cold, moist skin, often described as "cold and clammy."
4. Profuse sweating.
5. Pale skin color that may turn to bluish (cyanosis).
6. Shallow, labored, and rapid breathing that may become irregular or gasping.
7. Dilated pupils and dull lusterless eyes.
8. Marked thirst.
9. Nausea and vomiting.
10. Slowly, but steadily falling blood pressure. It is best to assume that anyone with a systolic blood pressure of 100mm Hg. or lower is developing shock.
11. Loss of consciousness in the late stages of severe shock.

Shock is a medical emergency and must be treated before further examination or first aid treatment can be performed. The following actions must be applied whenever the symptoms of shock are present.

1. Assure that the patient has an open airway and is breathing well.
2. Control bleeding with direct pressure and apply a tourniquet if necessary.
3. Place the patient in the prone position and elevate the lower extremities about 12 to 18 inches. Note: Avoid raising the legs further as this may inhibit breathing.
4. Calm the patient and avoid rough handling.
5. Keep the patient warm by placing blankets over and under them, but avoid overheating.
6. Splint fractures to lessen bleeding and minimize pain.
7. Do not give the patient anything to eat or drink.
8. Monitor the patient's level of consciousness, blood pressure, and other vital signs.
9. Get the patient to professional medical care as soon as possible.

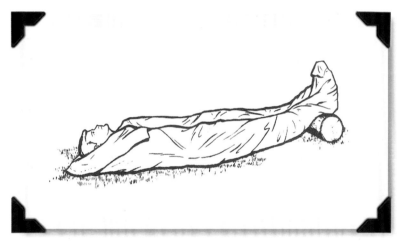

Patients in or going into shock are placed in the shock position with legs elevated 12 to 18 inches and covered with a blanket.

Compensated vs. Decompensated Shock

When blood volume first begins to drop, the body attempts to maintain blood pressure and organ profusion by increasing the heart rate and constricting the blood vessels. The signs of early, compensated shock include anxiety, rapid heartbeat, paleness, thirst, weak pulse, and a narrowing of the range between systolic and diastolic blood pressure. The patient's mental state and apparent condition may seem normal, but unless immediate steps are taken, decompensated shock will follow.

Decompensated shock develops when the body can no longer maintain sufficient blood pressure to sustain the vital organs. In short: the patient is dying. The systolic blood pressure falls below 90 mm Hg. Breathing becomes labored and weak, pupils dilate, the skin becomes ashen or cyanotic, and the level of consciousness declines. Finally, the patient becomes colder and loses consciousness. Unless professional care such as high-flow oxygen, IV fluids, and blood transfusions are available, the patient will die.

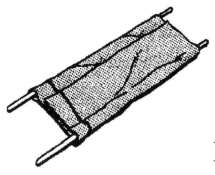

CHAPTER 11
HEAD INJURIES

Head injuries can range from superficial cuts and bumps to major damage to the brain, spine, and airway. In all cases of impact, or blunt force trauma (vehicle crashes, falls, assaults, etc.), it should be assumed that spinal injury may have occurred. Injuries to the face, nose, and jaw may create airway obstructions. Brain injury may have occurred even if there is no external sign of injury. Once the airway is assured, the cervical (neck) spine must be stabilized to prevent movement and potential damage. The patient's level of consciousness must be established and reassessed to detect potential brain injury. Damage to the brain and spinal cord can cause altered breathing patterns and respiratory insufficiency.

Spinal Immobilization

In any case where the patient is found unconscious after a fall, impact, or other potential head injury, the cervical spine should be immobilized immediately. Have someone hold the head in the neutral (face up and centered) position with very gentle traction, while the first aider assesses the airway and performs a full examination. In all cases where there is potential for a spinal cord injury, the jaw thrust method of opening the airway should be used in place of the head tilt/chin lift method. The first aider places the fingers behind the angle of the jaw and lifts it forward without significantly bending the spine backward. Then use the thumb to pull the patient's lower lip downward to permit breathing through the mouth as well as the nose.

Indications of brain injury include the following:

1. Deteriorating level of consciousness is the most significant sign of a brain injury.
2. Unequal pupil size and reaction to light.

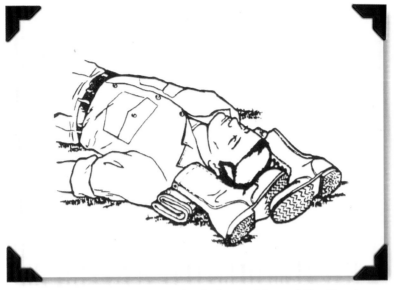

This "military expedient" method of spinal immobilization is just one example. Anything that keeps the head from turning will work.

3. Distended abdomen and little chest movement, indicating that the chest muscles may be paralyzed.

4. Low blood pressure below the injury when there is no evident blood loss, indicating dilated blood vessels.

5. Increasing blood pressure combined with slowing pulse indicates intracranial bleeding.

6. Conscious patient's inability to feel or move extremities.

7. Unconscious patient's failure to react, grimace, or withdraw when the first aider gently pinches the skin on the legs, abdomen, thorax, and face.

8. Nausea and vomiting are often a result of intracranial bleeding.

9. Altered breathing patterns.

10. Cyanosis (bluing skin) is a late finding that indicates significant brain injury.

Concussions

A concussion may result from a blow to the head. In some cases, a concussion may result in temporary unconsciousness. The patient may be confused or even not remember the event that caused the concussion. Most people recover from a concussive state rapidly. If the patient does not have a clear memory of the event or complains of dizziness, weakness, or vision changes, a concussion must be suspected. The patient should be closely monitored for several hours for declining level of consciousness and other signs of a more severe brain injury.

Intercranial Bleeding

The brain fills most of the intercranial space and has little room to move. An injury to the brain at the site of the impact is referred to as a coup injury. A countercoup injury to the brain may occur on the side opposite to the impact site as the brain bounces back against the interior of the skull. Coup-countercoup brain injury is common in vehicle collisions. Severe injury can result in laceration of blood vessels in the brain or in the meninges that covers the brain resulting in intercranial bleeding. Since there is little space around the brain, blood accumulates and exerts pressure on the brain. If the bleeding is severe the patient's mental state and level of consciousness may deteriorate rapidly. If progressive deterioration of awareness and level of consciousness is observed in a head injury patient, they require immediate access to professional care and probably surgery. Intracranial bleeding may also occur more slowly over several days. Constant monitoring is required and access to medical care is imperative at the first signs of deterioration. Any patient who has lost consciousness, regardless of other signs or degree of recovery, must be taken to an emergency room for professional evaluation. Increasing blood pressure combined with a slowing pulse rate is a reliable sign of head injury.

Skull Fractures

A skull fracture usually indicates the potential for serious brain injury. Signs of a skull fracture include the following:

1. Deformity or indentations of the skull upon palpation
2. Bruising around the eyes known as "raccoon eyes"
3. Bruising behind the ears known as "battle signs"
4. Pink, watery cerebral spinal fluid dripping from the nose and mouth

Do not attempt to pack the site of leaking cerebral spinal fluid as this may cause further brain damage. If cerebral spinal fluid is leaking from an open scalp wound it can be covered with a loose sterile dressing. Any impact severe enough to cause a skull fracture may also have caused spinal injury. Spinal immobilization, protection of the skull, and rapid access to professional care are critical.

Contusions

A severe impact may result in a contusion to the brain, causing the brain itself to swell within the skull and cause potential permanent or life-threatening damage to the brain. Brain contusions will produce all of the signs of brain damage, including altered levels of consciousness, numbness, weakness, and dilated pupils. While the first aider cannot assess or treat a brain contusion, the potential must be considered for all impact-related head injuries.

Lacerations

Laceration to the face and scalp are treated as any other soft tissue injury. Typical techniques for dressing head wounds are illustrated below.

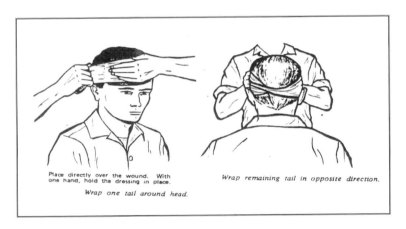

Place directly over the wound. With one hand, hold the dressing in place.

Wrap one tail around head.

Wrap remaining tail in opposite direction.

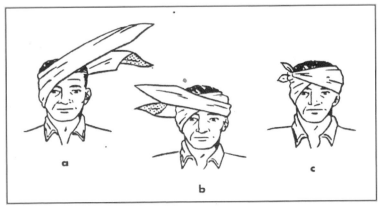

a

b

c

Nose Bleeds

Nose bleeds can result from facial injuries, a fractured skull, high blood pressure, or a sinus infection. Nose bleeds caused by a skull fracture should be treated by application of a dry, not too tight, sterile dressing. Most nose bleeds from other cases can be treated as follows:

1. Keep the patient calm and quiet.
2. Place the patient in a sitting position with the head tilted forward to prevent swallowing and aspiration of blood.
3. Apply pressure by pinching the nostrils and/or by placing a roll of 4 x 4 gauze between the gums and the upper lip.
4. If available apply ice over the nose to slow circulation.

Some nosebleeds originate further back in the nasopharynx and cannot be controlled by these methods. If the bleeding cannot be stopped by these methods, prompt access to professional care is necessary to prevent the development of hypovolemic shock

Patient Positioning

While patients exhibiting the signs and symptoms of shock are transported with their feet elevated, patients with potential intracranial bleeding should be transported with the head end of the board or stretcher elevated six inches to reduce intracranial pressure. In all cases of head injury, spinal immobilization must be sustained throughout evaluation, care, and transport.

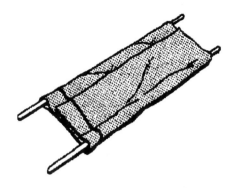

CHAPTER 12
EYE INJURIES

While injures to the eye or eyes may be concerning and cause agitation to the patient, they are never life-threatening. Unless the first aider can be sure that the eye injury is the only possible injury, a full examination and vital signs should be performed before assessing and treating the eye injury. Assessment of an eye injury must be performed with great care so as not to aggravate the injury and cause pain and even loss of vision. When examining for a potential eye injury look for the following:

1. Swollen or lacerated eyelids
2. Obvious penetrations of the eye
3. Bright redness of the lower eyelid (conjunctiva)
4. Redness of the corona (white) of the eye
5. Foreign objects on the eye surface
6. Blood collecting inside of the eye (hyphemia)
7. Unequal pupil size and reaction
8. Patient complains of pain and double vision
9. Ask the patient to follow your finger movement with their eyes. The eyes should move smoothly and equally together.
10. Protrusion or bulging of one or both eyes usually indicates serious head injury.

Foreign Objects in the Eye

Even a small foreign object such as a grain of sand or small debris will cause significant irritation and inflammation to the eye and conjunctiva. The first option is to flush the object out of the eye using a reliable eyewash solution or normal saline solution or sterile water. Always flush with the patient's head tilted so that the solution flows away from the nose and the other eye. The object may have caused some continued, temporary irritation after the object is gone. Objects that are stuck to the underside of the eyelid or the conjunctiva may not wash out. You can pull down the conjunctivae to reveal objects there and remove them with a soft, moist cotton-tipped applicator. The eyelid can be lifted by the eye lashes to reveal any object there and remove it with a soft, moist cotton-tipped applicator. Do not attempt to remove objects stuck to or in the corona, as this should be done by a professional.

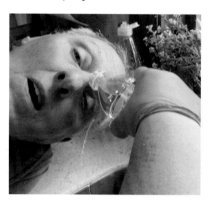

Use copious water to flush particles or chemicals from the eye. Tilt the head to prevent flushing into the opposite eye.

Lacerations to the Eye

Bleeding from a lacerated eye may be profuse; however, exerting pressure on the eye may squeeze out the various humors, causing permanent damage to the eye. Never exert pressure on the eye in any way. If part of the eyeball is exposed apply a moist sterile dressing to prevent it from drying. Cover the injured eye with a cup or other means that does not apply pressure, then cover the uninjured eye with a soft bandage. Transport to professional care as soon as possible to prevent vision loss.

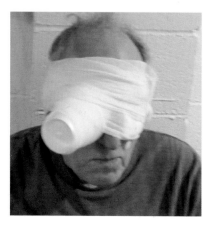

The cup over the eye can be used to isolate an impaled object in the eye or an eyeball that has been avulsed from the eye socket.

Blunt Force Trauma to the Eye

Impacts to the eye or the bones around the eye can cause bleeding into the eye and damage to the muscles and bones that support the eye. Bleeding into the interior of the eye can be observed, and the patient may complain of double vision and significant pain. A soft, no pressure cover should be placed over the eye and adjoining injured area, and the other eye should be covered to limit eye movements. Transport to professional care as soon as possible to prevent vision loss.

Impaled Objects in the Eye

An impaling object such as a nail or piece of glass stuck in the eye presents a significant challenge to the first aider. The object should never be removed in the field and cannot be stabilized as the eye will continue to move. Do not touch the eye or the object. Carefully cover the eye and impalement with a paper cup large enough to ensure that it does not contact the impalement. Cover the other eye to prevent movement and transport to professional care immediately.

Chemical Burns to the Eye

Chemical burns to the eyes can result from accidental splashing of corrosive liquids, deliberate assault, or exposure to various chemical agents such as pepper spray or teargas. Regardless of the source or the agent, the only treatment is immediate and copious flushing of the eyes with water or sterile saline solution. You cannot overirrigate. Flush the eye for at least twenty minutes or more. Be sure that the head is turned and the patient is positioned so that the flushed material flows away from the eyes and the mouth. After flushing, cover the eye or eyes with soft clean dressing and get the patient to professional medical care.

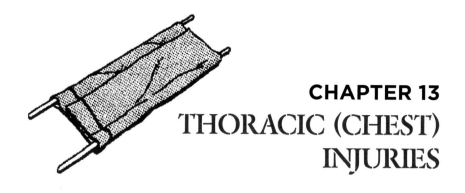

CHAPTER 13
THORACIC (CHEST) INJURIES

Because the heart, lungs, and great blood vessels are in the chest cavity, any injury to this area must always be considered as potentially life threatening. Chest injuries can be either open or closed. Closed injuries are those where the skin is not broken and are usually the result of blunt force impact such as being struck with a bat or impacting with a steering wheel. Open chest injuries can result from a knife, a bullet, or similar penetration. They can also be the result of broken ribs penetrating the skin.

Signs of Chest Injury

1. Pain at the site of the injury. This pain is often accompanied by painful breathing.
2. Discoloration (bruising) at the site of the injury.
3. Difficulty breathing. Breathing may be rapid and shallow in excess of 24 breaths per minute.
4. Failure of both sides of the chest to expand equally and normally.
5. Pale or bluish pallor to the skin, indicative of poor oxygen profusion.
6. Rapid and weak pulse and low blood pressure. These are signs of shock, indicative of significant internal bleeding
7. Coughing up blood. This usually indicates that a lung has been lacerated.

Care of Chest Injuries

Regardless of the cause or nature of the chest injury encountered, the same basic care priorities apply.

1. Maintain an open airway.

2.   Position the patient to best facilitate breathing and comfort. Patients who breathe better in a sitting position should be allowed to do so.
3.   Cover open chest wounds with sterile dressing.
4.   Control bleeding from chest wounds with manual direct pressure.
5.   Seal open, sucking chest wounds with occlusive dressings or other non-porous material.
6.   Stabilize impaled objects with extra bulky dressings around the object. Never remove an impaled object.
7.   Get patient to a hospital as fast as possible.

Rib Fractures

Fractured ribs are commonly caused by impact blows. The fifth through the tenth rib are the most commonly fractured. The patient can often point to the exact spot of the facture. A patient with multiple rib fractures will often lean towards the injured side with a hand over the fractures to splint the fracture and reduce the pain. Deep breathing is usually painful. Rib fractures usually do not require splinting, but in cases of multiple rib fractures, a sling and swath can facilitate comfort. Swathing should not be so tight as to inhibit breathing. It is important to be aware that a fractured rib may penetrate the lung or the chest wall, leading to hemothorax or pneumothorax.

Flail Chest

Flail chest develops when two or more ribs are fractured in two or more places. When this happens, the chest wall at that location becomes a free-floating segment that moves independently of the rest of the chest. The segment will collapse inward slightly when the chest expands and protrude upward slightly when the chest contracts. This condition is called paradoxical motion, or flail chest. This is a serious injury and is also very painful. The force required to create a flail chest will always cause damage to the lung tissue beneath the flail segment, resulting in swelling and bleeding into the lung and associated loss of lung function. This is a serious, life-threatening injury. The flail segment can be splinted by application of a pillow or similar material held firm over the segment, either held in place by the patient or secured with bandaging. The patient should be transported lying on the injured side so as to facilitate breathing by the uninjured lung.

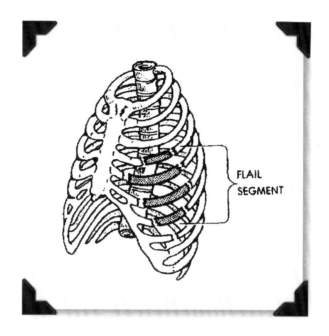

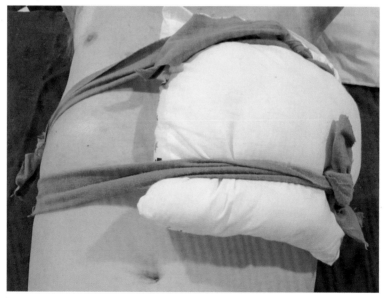

A pillow is used as a splint for a flail chest segment. The victim is then turned onto the injured side to improve respiration.

Pneumothorax

When air enters the pleural cavity outside of the lung, it is called a pneumothorax. The air separates the lung from the inside of the chest wall and collapses it towards the opposite side. This condition can be caused by air leaking into the pleural space from outside through a hole in the chest or from inside through a hole on the lungs. As the lung collapses its capacity is reduced. If this condition continues, the air will begin to shift the lung on the opposite side, further reducing lung capacity. As the degree of pneumothorax increases, hypoxia will develop. If the patient has an open wound to the chest, the degree of pneumothorax and hypoxia can be reduced by sealing the wound with an occlusive (non-porous) dressing. In the case of a closed or tension pneumothorax, where the air cannot escape, severe hypoxia will develop rapidly unless a needle decompression is performed to relieve the pressure.

Sucking Chest Wounds

An open pneumothorax, or sucking chest wound, results from a penetration of the chest wall from a sharp object such as a knife, bullet, or

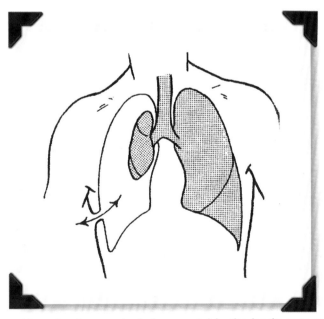

In a sucking chest wound, air from outside the body enters the chest cavity and compresses the lungs with each breath. Closing the hole will usually prevent further collapse. Vented chest seals allow some decompression.

flying debris. As the patient breathes and the chest expands and contracts, air will pass through the wound into the chest cavity instead of the lung. The lung will collapse further and further and the patient's ability to breathe will deteriorate unless the hole is sealed with an airtight dressing such as aluminum foil, plastic, vaseline, gauze, or a purpose-made chest seal device. The seal should be large enough to assure that it is not sucked into the wound, and it should be secured to the chest with tape. The patient's breathing must be monitored constantly. In some cases, a tension pneumothorax may develop after sealing the wound. If the patient begins to show symptoms of a tension pneumothorax remove the seal immediately.

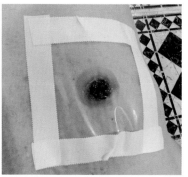

Any kind of airtight material can be used to seal a sucking chest wound, including Vaseline, gauze, plastic, or purpose-made seals. If a tension pneumothorax develops, the seal must be immediately removed.

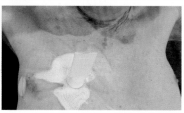

This Ashman™ seal has a one-way valve to vent excess air out of the chest. The valve and gauze is in the center of the round, adhesive, transparent seal.

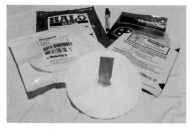

A variety of chest seal devices are available and at least two should be included in every trauma kit.

Tension Pneumothorax

A closed tension pneumothorax can develop as the result of an impact sufficient to rupture a lung, or from a broken rib penetrating a lung. A spontaneous pneumothorax can even just happen from normal breathing. In any case the signs and symptoms will be the same and the necessity for decompression will also be the same. In a tension pneumothorax the air cannot escape from the chest cavity, and therefore increases the pressure with each breath. The injured lung collapses to the size of a small ball and shifts towards the uninured lung, causing it to collapse. Pressure on the heart and great vessels will rapidly reduce the heart's ability to function. Death will result unless the pressure is relieved.

Signs of a Tension Pneumothorax

1. Severe respiratory distress
2. Falling blood pressure
3. Weak pulse
4. Bulging tissue in the chest and above the clavicle
5. A shift in the trachea away from the injured side
6. Cyanosis

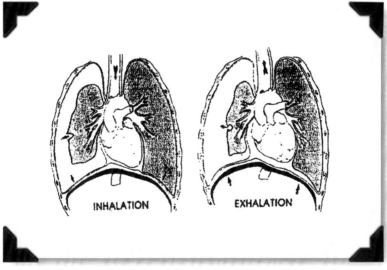

In a tension pneumothorax, the air outside the lungs collapses the lung more and more with each breath

Chest Needle Decompression

Needle decompression is an invasive procedure that goes beyond ordinary first aid and is normally performed by trained paramedics. Only if (1) the obvious signs of a tension pneumothorax are present, and (2) no immediate access to an emergency room or ambulance can be anticipated, should a first aider attempt this procedure.

1. Use a 14-gauge needle with a catheter three or four inches in length. Needles made specifically for chest decompression are sold online and should be included in advanced first aid kits.
2. Locate the space between the second and third rib, halfway between the sternum and the side (mid clavicle line) on the injured side.
3. Prepare of the site insertion with alcohol or anti-microbial scrub if time permits.
4. Insert the needle slowly, at a 90-degree angle over the top of the third rib into the second intercostal space.
5. Stop insertion of the needle once you hear the hissing of escaping air. There will be a distinct "pop" as you enter the chest cavity and relieve the pressure.
6. CAUTION: Extreme caution must be taken to avoid over-insertion of the needle as it may penetrate a lung or heart or major vessels.
7. Hold the catheter in place while removing the needle.
8. Secure the catheter in place with tape.

Needle decompression is a temporary lifesaving procedure. The victim will need to access professional medical attention as soon as possible.

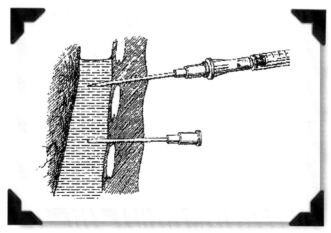

Position and depth of chest decompression needles.

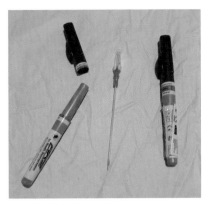

Decompression needles with catheters are available from survival supply and emergency medical vendors.

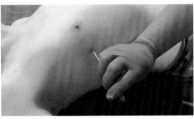

The needle is inserted until the air or blood is released. The needle is extracted, and the catheter remains in place.

Hemothorax

Hemothorax is the accumulation of blood in the chest cavity and frequently accompanies pneumothorax. The blood together with air accumulates in the pleural space and collapses the lung just as air does

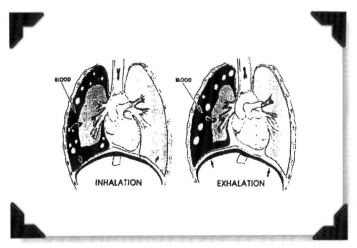

In a hemothorax, it is blood that fills the chest cavity and collapses the lungs. It may also be a combination of blood and air, but needle decompression will drain both.

in a pneumothorax, with the added complication of severe internal bleeding. The patient will exhibit many of the signs of pneumothorax combined with those of severe bleeding and shock. There is not much that the first aider can do beyond treating the pneumothorax and shock and getting the patient to professional care with all haste.

Other Complications of Chest Injury

Blunt force injuries may not cause pneumothorax, flail chest, or other obvious injury but can cause pulmonary contusion, causing blood to ooze into the lungs and interfere with the ability to exchange oxygen and carbon dioxide. Blunt force to the chest can also bruise the heart muscle itself and cause an irregular or paused beating. Irregular or paused heart rhythms can lead to heart failure and death. In extreme cases, blood and fluids may leak into the sack surrounding the heart. As the heart is compressed, the range between the systolic and diastolic blood pressure readings narrows, and the heart sound becomes muffled. The pulse becomes weak, and the veins in the neck become distended. This is a life-threatening medical emergency.

Finally: any chest injury can also result in damage to the pulmonary arteries, pulmonary veins, or inferior or superior vena cava. Bleeding from these major vessels into the chest cavity can result in the rapid onset of shock and death. The bottom line for chest injuries is that they can all be serious. Rapid assessment, effective treatment, and rapid access to professional care are essential to the patient's survival.

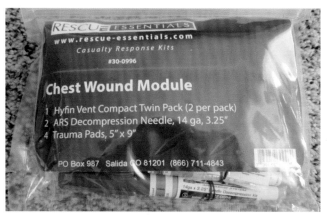

This chest wound module from Rescue Essentials™ has everything needed to treat a sucking chest wound or tension pneumothorax.

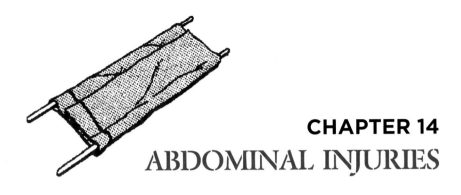

CHAPTER 14
ABDOMINAL INJURIES

The abdomen is the space below the diaphragm and ribcage. This space contains the stomach, intestines, liver, kidneys, bladder, gallbladder, and spleen. The aorta and inferior vena cava run through this space as well. Blunt and penetrating injuries to the abdomen can damage vital organs resulting in severe bleeding and life-threatening complications. The abdominal cavity can hold enough blood to cause shock and death without any sign of external bleeding. Rupture of hollow organs spilling the contents into the abdominal cavity can cause peritonitis, a severe inflammation of the peritoneum resulting in intense pain, muscular rigidity, and abdominal distention.

Evaluation of Abdominal Injuries

Permit the patient to lie prone or with the knees flexed and supported for comfort while conducting the examination for these signs. Most patients with severe abdominal injury or illness will prefer to lie still with the knees drawn up.

Signs and symptoms of abdominal injury include the following:

1. Local or general abdominal tenderness.
2. Abdominal bruising.
3. Resistance to movement due to pain.
4. Obvious wounds. A penetrating wound such as a gunshot wound may have a small entrance wound and a much larger exit wound. Be sure to check for exit wounds.
5. Evisceration of internal organs through the abdominal wall.
6. Altered vital signs such as rapid shallow respirations, declining blood pressure, rapid pulse, and other signs of shock.
7. Distention of the abdomen. Pulsing of the abdomen may indicate severe internal bleeding.
8. Nausea and vomiting as a result of damaged or ruptured internal organs.

Treatment of Blunt Abdominal Wounds

Blunt force–caused abdominal wounds may cause severe injuries to vital organs, ruptured or torn major arteries or veins, and intra-abdominal hemorrhaging. Be especially alert for signs of shock such as sweating, paleness, rapid pulse, and falling blood pressure. The patient should be positioned on one side with the head turned to one side to prevent aspiration of vomit. Keep the patient's mouth free of vomit and maintain a clear airway. Gain access to professional medical care without delay.

Treatment of Open Abdominal Wounds

Unless the wound is obviously superficial, the first aider should assume that the penetration has injured internal organs and major blood vessels even if the signs and symptoms have not yet presented. If the penetrating object is still in place, it should be left in place and stabilized with bulky dressings. Be sure to inspect thoroughly for exit wounds opposite of the entry point. Dry sterile dressing should be applied to all open abdominal wounds.

Treatment of Eviscerated Abdominal Wounds

When the abdominal wall is lacerated, abdominal organs may protrude through the wound. In some cases, a significant amount of

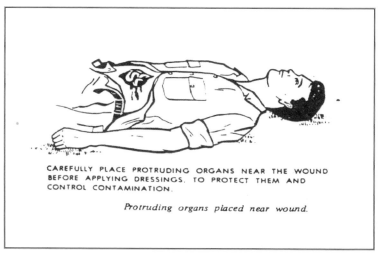

CAREFULLY PLACE PROTRUDING ORGANS NEAR THE WOUND BEFORE APPLYING DRESSINGS. TO PROTECT THEM AND CONTROL CONTAMINATION.

Protruding organs placed near wound.

A laceration to the abdomen can result in the intestines spilling out. A lot more intestines than shown here may spill out.

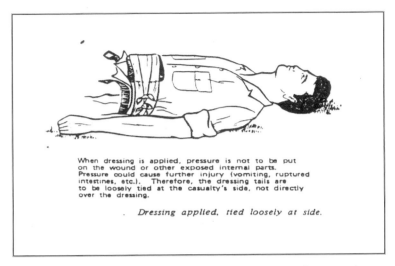

When dressing is applied, pressure is not to be put on the wound or other exposed internal parts. Pressure could cause further injury (vomiting, ruptured intestines, etc.). Therefore, the dressing tails are to be loosely tied at the casualty's side, not directly over the dressing.

Dressing applied, tied loosely at side.

All intestines must be placed on the abdomen and covered with a soft, moist dressing. The dressing must be kept moist to prevent the intestines from drying out.

the intestines may spill from the wound. The first aider should not attempt to push or replace the organs into the wound. The protruding organs must be kept moist and warm. Cover the organs with a moist, preferably sterile dressing. Keep the dressing moist with sterile water as needed. Aluminum foil securely taped over the wound can retain moisture and heat. Transport an evisceration patient in a prone position to prevent shifting of the organs.

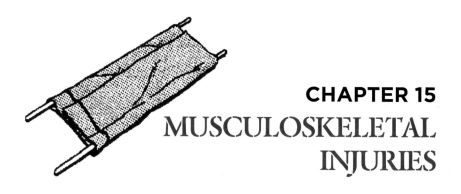

CHAPTER 15
MUSCULOSKELETAL INJURIES

Musculoskeletal injuries occur from violent trauma such as falls, collisions, and impacts. Damage to the musculoskeletal system includes strains, sprains, dislocations, and fractures. These types of injuries are common under normal conditions and even more frequent in disaster situations. It is important that the first aider be able to recognize and treat these injuries promptly and effectively to prevent further damage and potential disability.

Strains occur when the muscle is over-stretched or torn, but there is no damage to ligaments or joints.

Sprains are joint injuries in which the joint is partially or temporarily dislocated, and the supporting ligaments are stretched or torn.

Dislocations happen when the bone ends are completely separated at the joint (elbow, shoulder, knee, wrist, etc.), accompanied by tearing of the joint ligaments.

Dislocation Fractures are twin injuries that include the fracturing of the bone adjoining the dislocated joint.

Fractures are complete breaks in a bone and are classified as closed or open fractures. **Closed fractures** are those that do not involve an open wound that exposes the broken bone. They may be displaced where the bone ends are separated and displaced, or non-displaced when the bone breaks, but the ends remain in place and aligned. **Open fractures** also known as compound fractures are fractures where there is a break in the overlying skin at the fracture point. The break can be the result of the jagged bone ends puncturing the skin from inside, or from the force of an object, such as a bullet that penetrated the skin from the outside and then caused the fracture. Open fractures are much more serious than closed fractures because of greater blood loss and the danger of infection. Access to professional care must be obtained without delay.

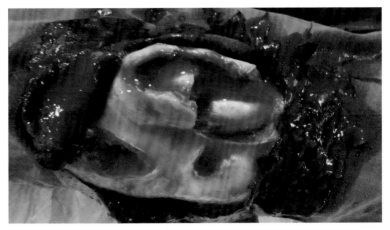

(Simulated) Open fracture with exposed bone ends. The wound must be bandaged without putting pressure on the bone ends, and the limb must be splinted as found prior to transportation.

Signs and Symptoms of Strains and Sprains

The signs and symptoms of strains are similar to those for sprains and even non-displaced fractures. The first aider should treat all musculoskeletal injuries as if they are fractures.

+ **Tenderness.** Tenderness over the site of the injury.
+ **Swelling.** Strains usually result in some tearing of blood vessels at the join, resulting in swelling.
+ **Inability to move.** In most cases the patient will guard the injured limb and joint and refuse to move it.

Signs and Symptoms of Dislocations

The joints most often dislocated are shoulder, elbow, hip, ankle, and fingers. The indications of dislocations are usually evident.

+ **Deformity.** Visible deformity at the joint.
+ **Swelling.** Swelling at and around the joint.
+ **Inability to move.** Complete loss of the ability to move the joint.
+ **Pain.** General pain and pain to the touch above the joint.

Signs and Symptoms of Fractures

+ **Deformity.** The injured extremity may be bent at an unnatural angle or rotated where no joint exists. If in doubt, compare the extremity to the opposite, uninjured one.

+ **Swelling.** While swelling may be indicative of any injury, it will always be present at a fracture site as the result of damage to the blood vessels. Swelling will develop rapidly after the injury and may be severe enough to mask any deformity. Swelling of the entire extremity will develop a few hours after the injury.

+ **Pain.** Tenderness and pain will immediately develop at the injury site. Gentle palpation of the site will reveal "point tenderness" over the fracture and is a highly reliable indication of an underlying fracture.

+ **Inability to move.** In most cases of fracture, the patient will refuse to move the injured limb and may hold or guard it against any movement. While guarding and the inability to move are reliable signs of a serious injury, the ability to move an injured extremity does not rule out a potential fracture. Non-displaced fractures are not always painful enough to prohibit movement, and the pain of other injuries may temporarily mask the pain from a fracture.

+ **False motion.** Movement of the extremity at points where motion does not normally occur is a positive sign of fracture, but movement should be avoided

+ **Grating.** Grating, also known as crepitus, caused by bone ends rubbing may be felt or heard as a grating sensation upon examination, but movement should be avoided

+ **Exposed bone fragments.** Visible bone ends or bone fragments in an open wound is an obvious indication of a fracture.

Evaluation of Musculoskeletal Injuries

Examination of musculoskeletal injuries can only begin after the patient's airway and breathing are established and any severe bleeding is under control. In all cases where severe or multiple musculoskeletal injuries are suspected, movement of the patient must be minimized and the potential for shock must be anticipated. While the patient may complain about one specific injury, the first aider must perform a thorough head-to-toe survey to locate all injuries. After determination of a musculoskeletal injury site, the first aider must assess the distal neurovascular function. This is to evaluate nerve function and blood circulation below the injury site.

+ **Pulse.** Palpate the radial (wrist) pulse for arm injuries and the posterior tibial (back of ankle) pulse for leg injuries.
+ **Capillary Refill.** Note the coloration of the finger and toenail beds. Pale or blue (cyanosis) indicates inadequate profusion. Gently pinch the fingertips. The color of the nails should recover, prompt and pink.
+ **Sensation.** The patient should be able to sense light touch to the fingers and toes distal to the injury.
+ **Motor function.** If the injury is above the hand or foot, have the patient attempt to wiggle the fingers or toes. If movement causes any pain, do not persist in movement. If the injury involves the hand or foot itself, do not request movement of finger or toes.

Principles of Splinting

1. When in doubt about the nature of the injury (bruise, sprain, fracture, etc.), splint it.
2. If possible, remove clothing from the extremity to be splinted to inspect the injury and secure the splint properly.
3. Cover all open wounds with sterile dressing prior to splinting. Avoid covering up bandaged wounds with splinting.
4. Do not move the patient before splinting.
5. Assess the distal pulse, circulation, sensation, and ability to move before and after splinting. If these functions are lost after splinting, loosen the splint, and gently reposition the limb to restore them before attaching the splint.
6. Whenever possible, splint any dislocation or fracture in the position it is found.
7. If the limb is so extremely deformed that it cannot be splinted as found, apply gentle traction to realign bone ends enough to splint.
8. Pad splints to prevent chafing and discomfort to the patient.
9. If possible, have one person hold and support the injured limb while another applies the splint. This will prevent movement and pain to the patient.

10. For bone fractures, the splint must immobilize the joint above and below the injury.

11. For joint injuries, the splint must extend to the bones on both sides of the injury.

12. Realigning a fracture may only be justified if no pulse, circulation, or sensation is detected below the injury; realign just enough to restore these functions.

13. Only if no access to medical facilities can be anticipated for an extended length of time can complete field realignment be justified. This requires at least two people. One person is required to apply (pull) firm, but gentle traction to the limb, while the other holds the limb and assesses the alignment. Ideally a third person should be holding the patient in place to prevent dragging. Once alignment is achieved, a rigid splint is applied and secured above and below the fracture before traction is removed.

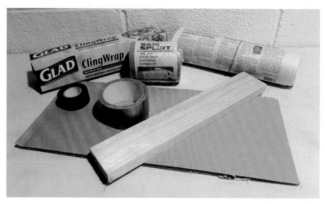

Cardboard, newspaper, or anything rigid can be used as a splint, held in place with cloth, tape, or even kitchen plastic wrap.

Splinting Methods

While following the above principles, all splinting is performed the same way regardless of the type of musculoskeletal injury involved. The objective is to immobilize the injury. While purpose-made splinting, such as a Sam Splint or an inflatable splint, are effective, the first aider can use wood, rolled newspapers, blankets, pillows, or even adjoining body parts (chest, opposite leg, etc.) to immobilize the injury. Cloth, tape, or other wide, strong material can be used to secure the splints in place. It doesn't have to be pretty; it just has to work. The following are some examples of splinting techniques.

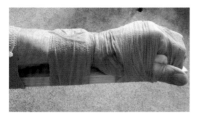

A fractured wrist needs to be splinted to immobilize the hand and forearm.

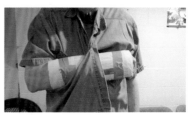

Expedient arm splint with buttoned shirt used as a sling.

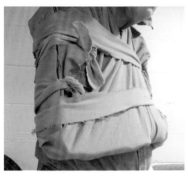

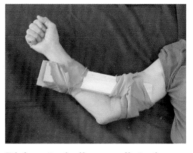

Dislocated elbow splinted as found. The same technique would apply to a knee joint.

Sling and swath method used for upper arm fracture. A Sam Splint is used for the splint, and torn cloth is used for the sling and the swathing.

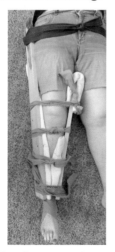

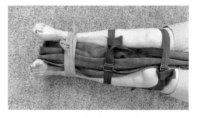

Lower leg splinted with blanket and the opposite leg as the primary splint.

Splinting for upper leg and hip fracture. Note the padding.

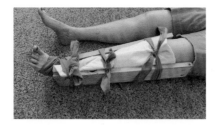

A well-padded splint of the lower leg and ankle.

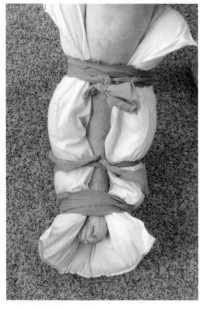

A pillow used as a soft-splint for a fractured or sprained ankle.

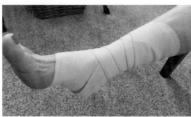

Ankle bandaged for sprain. Bandaging starts at the foot and crisscrosses upward. Elastic bandages are best for this.

Reduction of Dislocations

Dislocations occur when the bone ends are completely separated at the joint (elbow, shoulder, knee, wrist, etc.), accompanied by tearing of the joint ligaments. In addition to pain, dislocations will be evident by marked deformity at the joint. Dislocations are a common result of violent trauma such as vehicle crashes, falls, and assaults. Reduction of a dislocation should not be attempted by the untrained first aider unless access to professional care will be long delayed or the patient needs to regain function of the extremity to perform necessary survival activities. The most common dislocations are to the fingers, elbow, and shoulder.

REDUCTION OF A DISLOCATED FINGER

Finger dislocations are common injuries in many activities. A so-called jammed finger can be painful and render the associated hand useless. Furthermore, an unreduced finger dislocation can result in some permanent dysfunction if not reduced promptly.

1. Gently pull the finger until it returns to the natural alignment.
2. Splint the finger in the position of function, not rigidly straight.
3. The finger should be splinted in this position for three weeks to ensure adequate healing.

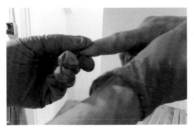 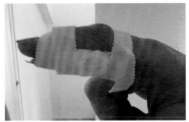

A dislocated finger can be reset by pulling until the joint realigns.

Fingers should be splinted in this "natural" position to retain functionality.

REDUCTION OF A DISLOCATED ELBOW

A dislocation to the elbow is particularly concerning because of the associated neurovascular bundle. Reduction should not be attempted if access to an orthopedic specialist will be available. An elbow dislocation may be indicated be the existence of a distinct, sharp point at the back of the elbow. Comparison to the back of the uninjured elbow should help the first aider verify this deformity.

1. The patient should be provided with pain medication if available.
2. The patient is placed on a high table, face down, as in the shoulder reduction method.

3. The upper arm is supported so that only the forearm hangs down.

4. Attach a 10-pound weight to the forearm as in the shoulder reduction method, or apply 10 pounds of manual pressure downward on the wrist while guiding the tip of the ulna back into position.

5. Sling and swathe the arm against the chest so that the elbow is at a 90-degree angle. Check the distal pulse. If the pulse is compromised, let the arm hang down a bit lower in the sling.

6. The elbow should be splinted (or cast) for at least three weeks and will require therapy and exercise to regain full function.

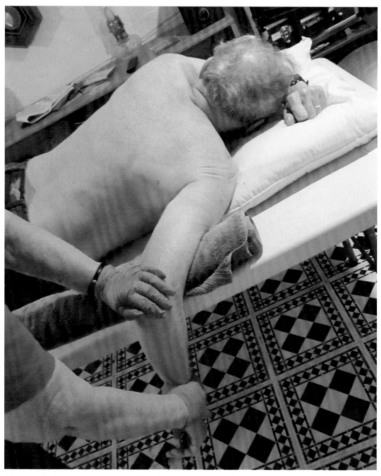

Patient lies on table with elbow extended. Gentle, downward traction is applied with one hand while the other hand guides the joint into place.

REDUCTION OF A DISLOCATED SHOULDER

Reduction of a dislocated shoulder should be performed as soon as possible, as pain and muscle spasms will intensify the longer the dislocation remains. The so-called "Stimson Maneuver" is the simplest and most effective method of reduction for a dislocated shoulder.

1. The patient lies face down on a high table, with the arm of the dislocation hanging over the edge.
2. The hanging forearm is wrapped in a wide cloth swath that extends below the hand.
3. A bucket of sand or water or a weight of about 10 to 15 pounds is attached to the end of the swath so that it pulls down on the arm.
4. In about twenty minutes the patient will be aware of a snap or clunk signifying that the joint has reset.
5. While the patient may be able to use the arm immediately, it is advisable place the arm in a sling and swath if possible.

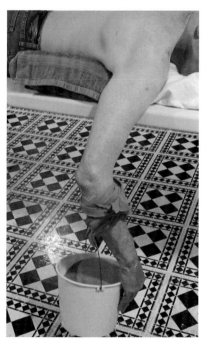

The patient is prone on a table with the whole arm extended downward. A bucket of water, or sand, or other weight of 10 to 15 pounds is attached the lower arm for traction. The joint will pop back into place after a few minutes.

Note: In all cases of field reduction of a dislocated joint, the joint should be reexamined by a doctor as soon as possible.

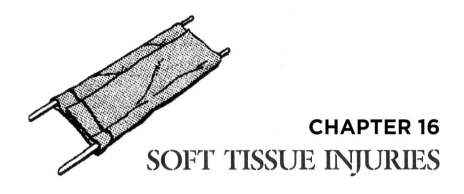

CHAPTER 16
SOFT TISSUE INJURIES

Soft tissue injuries are among the most common result of violent trauma, therefore bandaging and wound management are a core first aid skill. Once an airway, breathing, and circulation are established and any arterial bleeding has been controlled, the first aider can move on to locating and managing other injuries. There are two types of soft tissue injuries. Closed soft tissue injuries are those where the damage is below the skin, but the skin surface remains intact. Open wounds are those where there is a break in the skin surface.

Closed Soft Tissue Injuries

Closed soft tissue injures are usually the result of blunt force trauma that crushes the tissues, and damages blood vessels beneath the skin. Depending on the depth of the injury, varying amounts of fluids and blood will leak and accumulate beneath the skin. The buildup of fluids and blood will result in swelling, pain, and black or blue discoloration, generally referred to as bruising or ecchymosis. When larger blood vessels are damaged, a pool of blood may accumulate creating a "blood tumor" (hematoma). These can also occur due to fracture of a large bone such as the femur, or from organ damage. Large hematomas may indicate serious internal bleeding that may lead to shock, and should require immediate access to professional medical support.

First Aid for Closed Soft Tissue Injuries

Small bruises require no special attention. Subcutaneous bleeding can be reduced by the application of ice and local compression over the injury site immediately after the injury. Ice packs will cause the blood vessels to contract, reducing blood flow, while pressure will compress the vessels to help reduce bleeding as well. Elevation and splinting of the injured limb will also aid in reduction of bleeding and pain. The mnemonic for treatment of closed soft tissue injuries is ICES (ice, compression, elevation, splinting).

Open Soft Tissue Injuries

Open soft tissue injuries are openings in the protective layers of the skin resulting in bleeding and the potential for infection. There are four types of open soft tissue injuries.

Abrasions occur when the outer layer of the skin (epidermis) is damaged. Blood may ooze from capillaries in the lower (dermis) layer of the skin, but damage seldom goes deeper. These injuries are often referred to as "road rash" or "mat burns" and can be quite painful.

Lacerations are cuts caused by sharp objects. Depending on the cause these cuts may be smooth and straight or jagged. Lacerations penetrate into the subcutaneous tissues, and may go deep into the underlying muscles, nerves, and blood vessels.

Avulsions are injuries in which a section of skin is either torn entirely away or is left hanging as a flap of tissue. Avulsions usually involve tearing of the subcutaneous tissue from the lower muscle covering (fascia) and involve significant bleeding. If the flap remains attached by a significant area of skin, circulation to the tissue will sustain it, but if the attachment area is small or the flap is completely torn away, it will die if not reattached by medical professionals within a short time.

Punctures are holes in the skin caused by pointed objects such as knives, splinters, or bullets. External bleeding from puncture wounds is usually not significant, but wounds to deeper arteries and organs may result in severe bleeding and death. Puncture wounds may go completely through the body as a "perforated" or "through and through" wound. The first aider must always examine for an exit wound. Exit wounds can often be larger and more damaging than the entry wound.

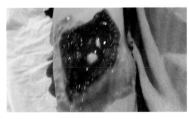

A very deep laceration wound exposing the bone will require professional care.

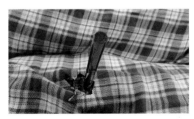

Impaled objects should not be removed unless they interfere with breathing.

First Aid for Open Soft Tissue Injuries

In order to effectively assess and manage any soft tissue injury, it is necessary to remove any clothing that covers the wound. It is usually best to cut away the clothing rather than try to remove it because the necessary movement may further the injury and aggravate pain and bleeding. The objectives of open soft tissue wound treatment are to control bleeding, prevent further contamination, and immobilize the injured part. Bleeding can be controlled by application of a sterile dressing that covers the entire wound. If bleeding continues, the original dressing should be left in place and additional dressings placed over it. When the bleeding is controlled, roller bandaging can be used to secure the dressings in place. If the injury is extensive, the injured extremity should be splinted to reduce bleeding. All open wounds will be contaminated to some extent by the source of the injury and the contaminants on the skin and clothing. In most cases the first aider should avoid trying to remove hair, clothing, and dirt from the wound, as this may worsen bleeding and pain. Application of a sterile dressing will prevent further contamination until the patient reaches professional medical care, where wound cleansing and debridement can be performed.

Bandaging Principles and Methods

While sterile, purpose-made bandaging products are preferred, the first aider may need to improvise. Bandaging may be created by tearing cotton material into long strips, usually two inches wide and three to four feet long. These bandages can be sterilized by boiling and drying, heating to 132 degrees Celsius (270 degrees Fahrenheit) for five minutes, or microwaving for no more than 60 seconds.

If no other bandaging materials are available, kitchen plastic wrap can be used, wrapped tightly around the entire extremity to cover the wound.

Self-adhesive and elastic bandages usually do not require additional methods to stay in place, but surgical tape may be necessary to secure cotton bandaging or gauze. If surgical tape is not available, electrical tape or duct tape can be used.

SECURING CLOTH BANDAGES

In the absence of tape, there are two methods for securing bandages in place after wrapping them around an extremity.

Tear the ends of the bandage lengthwise into two strips. Run one strip around the extremity in the direction of bandaging and the other back in the opposite direction and tie them together where they meet. If you have enough bandaging material after securing the dressing, make a large loop in the remaining material leaving a long free end. Bring the free end around and tie it into the loop.

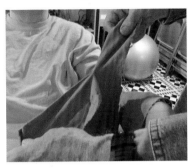

1 Tear the ends lengthwise, long enough to go around the limb in opposite directions.

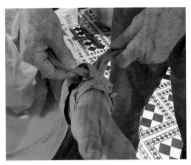

2 Bring around and tie over the wound.

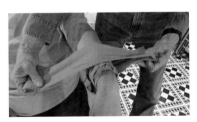

3 Make a big loop.

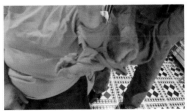

4 Bring the loop one way and the end the other way, then tie securely.

Whenever practical, have someone hold an extremity while you apply bandaging to prevent movement.

When winding a bandage around an extremity always start at the narrower, distal end of the limb.

If using non-self-adhesive bandaging it will be necessary to "lock" the starting end in place to prevent unwinding as you pull the bandage around the limb the first time around. Overlap a corner of the material and then wrap over the tab before continuing bandaging.

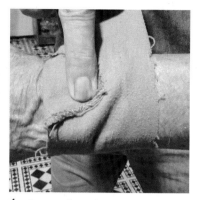

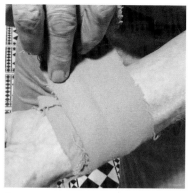

1 Start a bandage lock by folding over one corner.

2 Tightly wind over the tab and continue wrapping bandage.

CRAVAT BANDAGING

The techniques for bandaging various parts of the body using a cloth cravat are illustrated below.

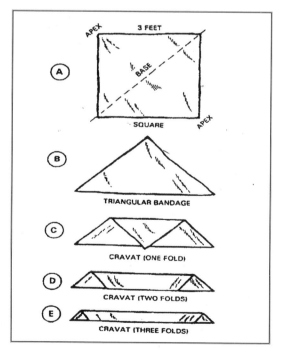

The basic three-foot-by-three-foot cravat can be used as a sling, folded into a triangular bandage or a cravat as shown above.

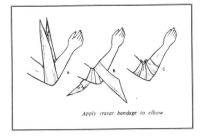

Apply cravat bandage to elbow.

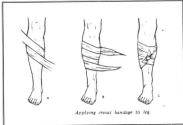

Applying cravat bandage to leg.

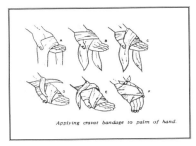

Applying cravat bandage to palm of hand.

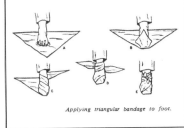

Applying triangular bandage to foot.

First Aid for Avulsions

When the flap of tissue is still attached, it should be carefully replaced into the original position and secured with a dry sterile dressing. If the avulsed tissue is completely detached, the tissue should be placed in sterile gauze inside a plastic bag and transported to the emergency room with the patient. Detached tissue can often be replanted if it is kept cool and dry and reaches professional care promptly.

First Aid for Impalements

Impalement occurs when an object has penetrated the body and remains in place. The following rules apply to first aid for any impalement.

Do not attempt to remove the object. Any movement may do further damage and cause additional bleeding. Apply direct pressure around the wound without moving the object. The only time that an impaling object can be removed is if it is obstructing breathing, such as through the jaw or cheek.

Use bulky dressings around the object to hold it in place. If the object is still fixed to a wall or other large immovable object, cut or saw it off while avoiding moving the object or the patient.

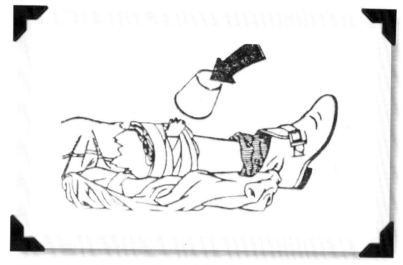

An impaled object must be stabilized with bulky dressings all around prior to transport.

The patient must be transported to an advanced care facility for removal of the object and necessary surgical repairs of the wound.

First Aid for Amputations

Amputations can be limited to a piece of tissue or can involve the separation of an entire limb. The objectives of first aid for amputations are to control bleeding and bandage the stump of the limb where the amputated part was severed. Treat the patient for shock and try to preserve the integrity of the amputated part so that reattachment in a hospital is possible. In cases of a clean amputation, severe bleeding may not occur immediately, but direct pressure and the application of a tourniquet above the amputation is still necessary to limit blood loss and reduce the severity of shock. The amputated extremity (tissue, finger, hand, and arm) must be wrapped in dry sterile dressings, placed in a plastic bag, and kept cool. Avoid over cooling, freezing, or soaking an amputated part as this may render reattachment impossible.

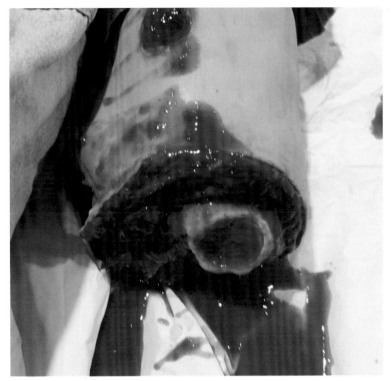

(Simulated) A limb amputation may or may not result in arterial bleeding. It will require sterile bandaging with or without a tourniquet and prompt transportation to the nearest ER with the retrieved body part.

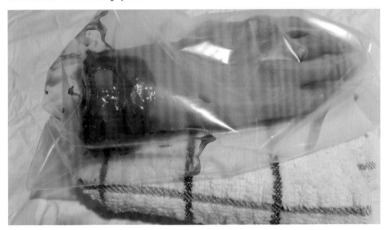

Severed body parts can be placed in plastic bags and kept cool with wrapped cold-packs. Do not let the part get wet or freeze as this will make reattachment problematic.

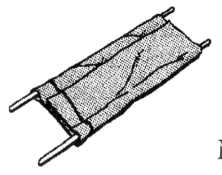

CHAPTER 17
WOUND MANAGEMENT AND CLOSURE

Management of deep wounds beyond immediate first aid should be performed by trained medical professionals in a clinical facility, but in the event of a large-scale disaster, professional care may be temporarily or indefinitely delayed. In the absence of antibiotics, infection and scarring are the major concerns. Healing is a natural process, but without effective closure it is usually slow and leaves greater scars than professionally closed wounds. There are two natural closure processes.

Primary Closure usually occurs to small, clean, incisions such as razor cuts and paper cuts, where the edges are clean and close together. Simple bandaging and disinfecting will be all that is required.

Secondary Closure or healing by secondary intention occurs when the wound edges are not even or close together, leaving a gap. In this case a granular tissue web will form across the opening to fill the gap between the edges. This process may take several weeks. The wound will weep and be open to infection until the tissue bridges the opening. Bandaging needs to change regularly. The initial tissue will be very delicate and should be protected for several weeks after forming. Scaring will usually be obvious and permanent.

Note: This author experienced several long, wide, and very contaminated wounds when no professional care was available. The open wound wept for several weeks, and I had to change soaked bandages several time a day, but they did heal, I still have the scars on my right knee. With good wound care, a good immune system, and a bit of luck nature can be amazing.

Managing Infected Wounds
The first aider should always be alert for the development of an infection in an open wound. Patients with weakened immune systems, poor circulation, malnutrition, or obesity are more inclined

to develop infections. Injuries sustained from dirty implements, in unsanitary environments, or from animal bites are highly inclined to become infected. Signs of an infection include:

1. Redness around the wound that may feel hot to the touch
2. Yellow pus oozing from the wound
3. Aches and pains
4. Malaise and fever
5. The redness may spread away from the wound site in streaks

If any of these signs develop, all efforts should be made to get the patient to professional care, as untreated infections can lead to loss of a limb or death. Complications can include an infection of deeper tissues known as cellulitis, a life-threatening blood infection known as sepsis, or necrotizing fasciitis, also known as the flesh-eating disease.

Mild antibiotic ointments (triple antibiotic) are available at pharmacies and should be kept at home and in first aid kits for shallow cuts and abrasions. Stronger antibiotics, marketed for animal wounds, can be obtained without prescription from farm supply stores. Animals tend to suffer cuts on barbed wire and other highly contaminated objects, so effective topical and internal antibiotics are available that can work just as well for human wounds. These antibiotics include amoxicillin, cephalexin, penicillin, clindamycin, doxycycline, and trimethoprim-sulfamethoxazole. These antibiotics can also be found at aquarium supply stores (for fish) and online from survival outfitters.

Wound Pain Reduction
All wounds are painful. Ordinary over-the-counter pain medications can help reduce pain. For bad pain, if prescription strength medications are available, use according to directions. One alternative is to combine two Tylenol (acetaminophen) tablets with three Advil (ibuprofen) tablets. Taken together these can provide pain relief comparable to codeine.

Wound Cleansing
Wound cleansing is usually performed by professional at a hospital, but in disaster situations or remote locations where professional care is not available or will be delayed, the first aider may need to perform this procedure. The purpose of this procedure is to remove foreign

matter and harmful bacteria from the wound before closure takes place. You may not get every particle, but the more you remove the more likely the body's natural defenses will be able to overcome an infection.

The most effective method of wound cleansing is water irrigation. While sterile water is preferred clean tap water can be used. A forceful stream can be created by using a squeeze bulb, a syringe, or by filling a plastic bag with water and poking a pinhole in it, then squeeze the bag to create a strong stream to flush the wound. Debridement is a more aggressive technique. In debridement physicians cut away the dead tissue at the edges of the wound, but this is not something the untrained first aider should attempt. Field debridement can approximate this procedure by vigorously scrubbing the area with clean gauze or cloth to remove bits of tissue and debris. This can be painful and will probably promote some bleeding so it should be done quickly. If tweezers or forceps are used to remove large debris, they must be sterilized by boiling for at least five minutes. Once cleansing and debridement is completed, cover the wound with a dry sterile dressing. Chemicals such as alcohol, hydrogen peroxide, or tincture of iodine should not be used on open wound because they damage the good flesh at the wound edges and inhibit healing.

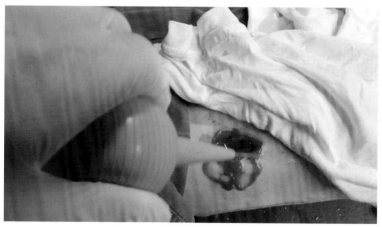

A bulb syringe is ideal for flushing deep wounds.

DAKIN'S SOLUTION

Battle statistics from the Civil War and World War I that show numbers of killed and wounded are misleading because a large percentage of the "wounded" died a few days or weeks later from septic wounds when there were no antibiotics available. Deep wounds are difficult to clean and are highly contaminated and ideal for biological growth. This can lead to the development of "gas gangrene." Gangrene is tissue death, and gas gangrene is a severe form caused by the clostridium perfringens bacteria or from Group A streptococcus. In deep wounds, the low oxygen conditions produce toxins that kill tissue. The use of Dakin's solution significantly reduced the development of infection and gangrene in deep wounds during World War I.

"Dakin's Solution" was an antiseptic fluid developed by a British chemist and a French-American surgeon. This was basically a 1/10 strength Clorox solution, with a little boric acid in sterile water. They would simply run the fluid over/through the wound. The solution would kill germs and dissolve dead tissue without harming healthy tissue. Studies indicate that solutions weaker than .025% are ineffective and stronger than .25% kill healthy tissue, so a .025%–.050% solution is recommended. The wound needs to be kept open and flushed frequently, as the solution remains effective for a short time on the wound. With the growing threat of antibiotic-resistant strains of staphylococcus and the possibility of shortages of antibiotics in a large-scale emergency, "Dakin's Solution" might be something to consider. In an emergency, one could make up the solution from available bleach and boric acid, but it can be purchased online for about sixteen dollars per sixteen-ounce bottle. Some doctors still prescribe Dakin's for wound care, so some pharmacists may have it.

Wound Closure Methods

Tight closure of deep wounds is not recommended in the absence of antibiotics as it is more likely to lead to the development of infection and gangrene. These methods can be used for clean shallow wounds or when there is adequate access to antibiotics.

BUTTERFLY BANDAGES

Butterfly bandages or Steri-Strips™ are the preferred method for wound closure. These devices can be applied quickly and adjusted or removed as needed. These bandages are simply strips of tape with a non-adhesive bridge in the center to bridge the wound. You apply one end of the tape to one side of the wound, then pull the bridge across the wound and secure the other end of the tape. You can use as many of these strips as necessary over the length of the wound. As with any wound closure method: just bring the wound edges to contact. Avoid pulling the edges tightly together so as to raise or pucker the wound as this will create an unsightly and permanent scar. Butterfly bandages and Steri-Strips may not hold on places such as knees and elbows where frequent bending takes place; in such locations, staples or sutures may be necessary.

Wound Closure Devices

An advancement over butterfly-type bandages are the purpose-made closure devices originally introduced by the Israeli military to replace suturing. Wound closure can certainly speed healing and reduce scaring, but the problems with suturing are:

✦ The needles and suturing material introduce additional infection sources and pain to the area.
✦ Suturing is often difficult on jagged wounds and under wet, dark conditions.
✦ If infection does develop, sutures are slow and hard to remove.
✦ Proper suturing requires training and constant practice.

The Israeli method uses a device that consists of two pieces that are stuck with adhesive to each side of the wound. A "zip tie"–like

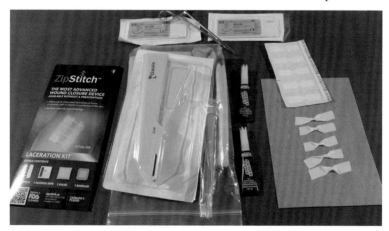

Wound closure devices, bottom left to right: ZipStitch™, stapler in package, two tubes of Super Glue, homemade and store-bought butterfly bandages. Top: sterile suturing needles and thread with needle holder.

cable is then put through these anchors and pulled until the wound is closed. You can line up as many of the anchors as necessary along the wound edges and close each one to achieve a long closure. A commercially available version of this device is the ZipStitch, which comes with an alcohol wipe, gauze, and bandage. Several of these in the first aid kit would provide an excellent alternative to sutures for deeper wounds.

SUPER GLUE

Super glue is an effective closure method for shallow, clean, and straight lacerations. Ordinary super glue sold in most hardware stores can be used to close wounds, but it does contain irritants and generates heat that can damage tissue. Purpose-made "medical glue" or veterinary glue such as Suri-Lock™ or Vet-Glu™ are better, if available. Do not use glue on facial wounds, wounds over joints, jagged wounds, deep wounds, puncture wounds, or dirty wounds.

Wound Closure with Super Glue

1. Be sure wound is clean and free of contaminants, and the wound edges are clean and dry.
2. Apply just enough glue to close the wound.
3. Just move the edges to contact. Avoid tenting the edges.
4. Hold the wound closed long enough for the glue to set.
5. Caution: Use care to avoid gluing your fingers to the wound.
6. Caution: Do not put too much glue on the wound, less is more.
7. Note: If a bit of blood gets into the glue it will not do any harm.
8. Note: If it is necessary to remove the glue (unlikely), use acetone (nail polish remover). It will sting but be effective.
9. Note: Wounds closed with super glue cause little or no scarring compared to other methods.

STAPLES

Stapling devices are handy and quick methods for wound closure. The disadvantages are that they are bulky in the first aid kit, a bit painful to apply, and punch additional holes in the skin. The Precise Five Shot™ by 3M is one such device. I still have a scar over my right eye from a stapled wound.

SUTURING

While proper suturing is considered the gold standard of wound closure, it is a difficult skill to master and must be practiced regularly to be maintained. A one-time suturing class will usually not be of much value two or three years later. Suturing is not advisable for deep wounds without access to effective antibiotics, as it will usually result in the development of infection and gangrene. The procedure is somewhat painful in the absence of topical anesthetics, and of course involves poking more holes in the skin. Suturing is not included in any first aid courses but is part of some "survival" medical classes. The Apprentice Doctor™ sells a suturing course training kit online that includes suturing instruments, materials, instructions, and artificial skin. One can acquire suturing kits from survival suppliers such as Nitro-Pack, or Rescue Essentials™. You can practice suturing using chicken breasts or pigs' feet.

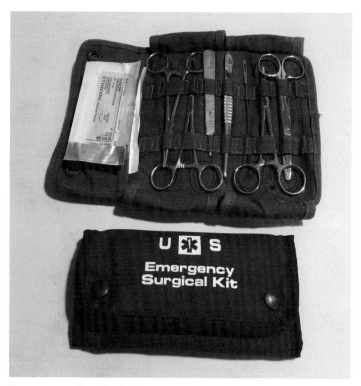

Emergency Surgical Kits contain everything needed to perform minor surgical procedures and suturing of wounds.

The following instructions are intended for informational purpose and should not be attempted without training and practice.

Steps for Simple Suturing

1. The wound should be cleansed prior to suturing. Disinfect the area around the wound with surgical scrubs or soap and water. Shave the area if necessary.
2. The needle should be inserted about 2- to 3-eighths of an inch (2–5 mm) from the edge of the wound, and sutures should be spaced approximately four per inch of wound length.
3. Grasp the needle holder firmly and lock the needle in place.
4. Push the needle so that it will pass directly through the skin with a twisting motion so that the needle will pass completely through the skin on one side of the wound, just through the epidermis, and cross the wound.
5. The needle should then be reinserted through the underside of the epidermis at about the same distance as the initial insertion from the wound edge and brought up through the skin surface.
6. Use forceps or fingers to even the wound edges.
7. Loop the suture around the needle holder once.
8. Grasp the short end and pull the wound closed, taking care not to pucker or overlap the wound edges.
9. Loop the long end around the needle holder again in the opposite direction to form a square knot.
10. Repeat the steps in the original direction to create a more secure knot.
11. Cut off the thread above the knot and repeat the suturing process until the wound is closed.
12. It may be advisable to cover the sutured area with a sterile dressing, but the sutures should be inspected regularly to observe for infections.

Steps In Suturing

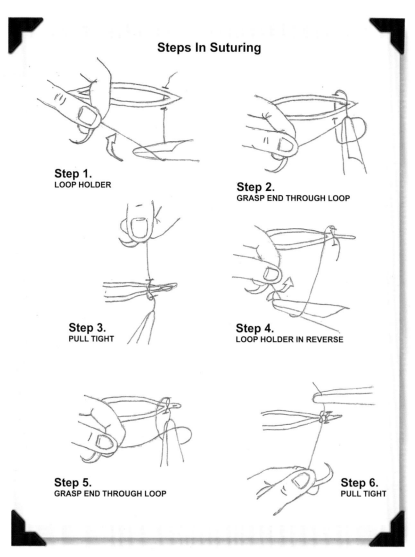

Step 1.
LOOP HOLDER

Step 2.
GRASP END THROUGH LOOP

Step 3.
PULL TIGHT

Step 4.
LOOP HOLDER IN REVERSE

Step 5.
GRASP END THROUGH LOOP

Step 6.
PULL TIGHT

The above illustrations show the procedure for suturing a wound using a needle holder.

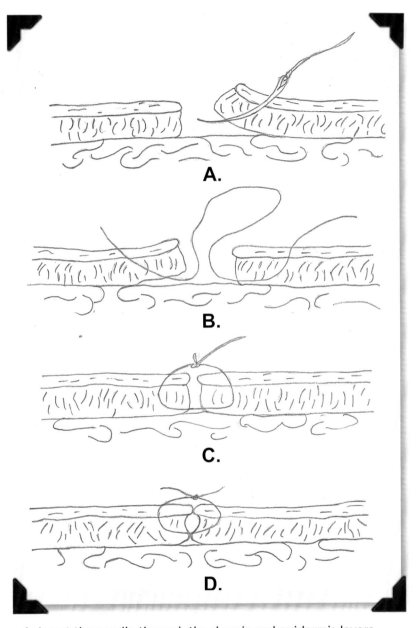

A: Insert the needle through the dermis and epidermis layers only. B: Bring the needle upward through the tissue on the opposite side. Make sure that the needle is drawn through the same depth and distance from the edges on both sides. C: Draw the edges together. D: Tie edges close enough to maintain contact but not so tight as to pucker and cause a raised scar.

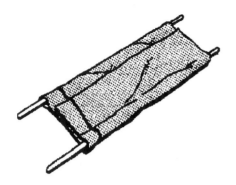

CHAPTER 18
BURNS

Burn injuries frequently occur from the immediate cause or secondary effects of a major disaster. Out-of-control forest fires are a normal occurrence in many regions. Civil disorder is often accompanied by arson. During power interruptions, citizens are often forced to use propane heaters, gasoline generators, alcohol stoves, kerosene lamps, and other sources of fire and burns. During emergencies, access to fire department and emergency medical services is often delayed or not available at all. Citizens should always have several large fire extinguishers on hand and be ready to administer first aid for burns.

Burn Classification

Burns are classified as first, second, or third degree depending on their depth into the body tissue.

First-degree burns are those in which only the outer part of the (epidermis) skin has been injured. The skin is reddened, but there are no blisters.

Second-degree burns go through the epidermis into the lower layers of the dermis, but not into the subcutaneous tissue. They are characterized by blistering and tend to be very painful.

Third-degree burns penetrate the dermis into the subcutaneous fat and beyond. Third-degree burns appear dry, leathery, brown, white, or charred. These burns may not be painful because the nerve endings have been burned away, but the area surrounding a third-degree burn usually will include second- and first-degree burns.

The seriousness of burns is a combination of the degree of the burn and the size of the body area that is burned. The method for classification of the burn area is "the rule of nines." The body surface area is divided into seven areas, each assigned a numerical percentage value of or divisable by nine as follows:

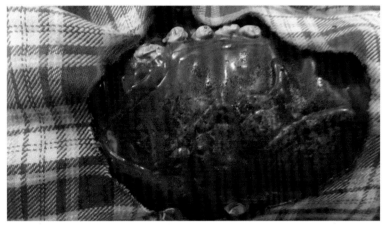

This (simulated) burn shows charred third-degree burns with blistered second-degree burns and surrounding first-degree burned tissue.

> The front of the torso = 18 percent
> The back of the torso = 18 percent
> Each leg, front and back = 18 percent
> Each arm, front and back = 9 percent
> The head, front and back = 9 percent
> The genitals = 1 percent

For example, the front of the torso and one leg would be a 36 percent burn.

Combining the percent of the body affected and the depth of the burns is used to determine the severity of the injury. Other factors in determination of significance of a burn injury are the age (very young or very old) of the patient and other injuries or health conditions.

Minor burns are classified as third-degree burns involving less than 2 percent of the body surface, or second-degree burns involving less than 15 percent of the body surface.

Moderate burns include any third-degree burns to more than 2 percent of the body, and second-degree burns covering more than 15 percent of the body. First-degree burns that involve from 50 to 75 percent of the body are also classified as moderate burns.

Critical burns are any third-degree burns that involve more than 10 percent of the body surface, and second-degree burns over more than 25 percent of the body. Any third-degree burns involving the hands, feet, face, or genitalia are to be considered critical. Burns that involve fractures or respiratory injuries must also be treated as critical.

For children, the burn classifications above can be elevated one level with burns considered moderate for adults being critical for children and all but very small burns classified as moderate.

First Aid for Thermal Burns

Preliminary first aid for burns is simple but must be initiated promptly to be effective.

1. Stop the burning process. In addition to putting out any burning clothing or debris, the first aider must cool the skin with cold water or cool wet dressing to stop the ongoing burning damage to deeper tissue.
2. Cut away burned clothing but avoid touching the burned area. Do not try to remove burned material from the burn.
3. Cover the burned area with dry sterile dressings to decrease the risk of infection.
4. Be alert to for signs of shock, airway obstruction, hypothermia, and other complications
5. Get the patient to medical care.

While ointments should not be applied to second- or third-degree burns, first-degree burns and surface chemical burns can be treated with Sulfadiazine 1 percent ointments. Sulfadiazine decreases the risk of bacteria causing blood infections. Prescription Sulfadiazine comes in 2 percent strength, but efficacy of the over-the-counter strength can be improved by covering the treated burn with plastic cling wrap.

Complications of Burns

Damage to the skin's capacity to protect the body from infection, retain bodily fluids, and regulate body temperature can result in severe, life-threatening complications. The first aider should be aware of the following:

1. Ointments and salves should never be used on any burns that exceed the "minor burn" classification.
2. While cooling with cold water can reduce the severity of a burn when immediately applied, it should not be sustained for more than ten minutes, to avoid over-cooling.

3. Infection is the greatest danger for third-degree burns; only clean water and sterile dressing should be used.

4. Extensive burns cause significant loss of fluids that can result in hypovolemic shock. Be prepared to treat the patient for shock.

5. Burned tissue is unable to regulate temperature, leading to the development of hypothermia. Keep the patient comfortably warm.

6. Burned tissues such as fingers and toes should never be bandaged together. Soft sterile dressing must be used to separate adjoining burned tissue to prevent it from healing together.

7. Any indication of burns to the face or potential inhalation of hot or toxic smoke or fumes creates the danger of respiratory compromise. Any patient with such indication, regardless of how minor the apparent burns may be, should be rushed to emergency care.

8. In the event that professional care is not available, first aid for burns must be directed at preventing infection, reducing pain, and maintaining patient hydration.

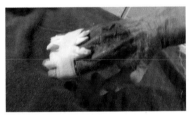 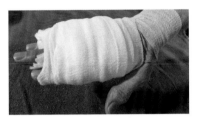

Never bandage burned tissue together. Soft, sterile gauze pads are used to separate these burned fingers.

Soft, sterile bandaging of burned hand.

Chemical Burns

Contact with corrosive chemical such as acids or alkalis can create serious burns. The primary action for the first aider is to stop the burning by massive flushing with water and removal of all clothing that may retain the corrosive substance. Care must be taken to avoid contacting or splashing of the corrosive onto the first aider or other persons. Wearing a face shield or goggles is particularly important to protect the eyes, and latex gloves should be worn to protect the hands while administering care. Flooding should be continued until the patient says that the pain has stopped, and then about ten minutes longer. If the first aider has become contaminated, all contaminated clothing must be removed and the underlying skin should be flushed. Be sure to identify the chemical involved so that you can tell the responding emergency care personnel.

Chemical burns to the face and eyes are always medical emergencies. Copious flushing of both eyes must be started immediately and sustained for at least fifteen minutes. Corrosive chemicals may have been ingested or inhaled leading to serious, life-threatening respiratory complications. All cases where corrosive chemicals have contacted the face or head must get to professional care immediately.

Extinguishing a Burning Victim

The first aider may encounter a person whose clothing is still on fire. This situation creates the potential for ever greater damage to the patient and a real hazard to the first aider. The standard procedure for extinguishing a burning person is "stop, drop, and roll." A person who is on fire may tend to run or thrash, but this may only cause the fire to increase. Command the person to stop, drop to the ground, and roll, to put the flames out. If the person fails to obey, it may be necessary to tackle the person and roll them. Alternatives include the following: beating the flames out with a jacket, wrapping the person in any available blanket or rug to smother the flames, or dousing the flames with water or a fire extinguisher. Once the flames are out, immediately cool the entire burned area with cold water or even snow if available. After ten minutes of cooling, the burned clothing can be carefully cut away, and dry sterile dressing can be applied.

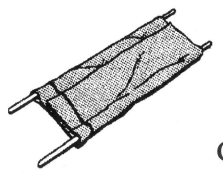

CHAPTER 19
HEAT AND
COLD INJURIES

The body operates within a narrow range of temperature. Any significant deviation up or down from the normal 98.6-degree Fahrenheit internal body temperature can create a domino effect of internal system failures, organ damage, and death. The body works to maintain the stability of body temperature through regulation of blood flow, sweating, shivering, and metabolism. When these methods are overwhelmed by an environment's excessive heat or cold conditions, hyperthermia (heat stroke) or hypothermia (exposure) can develop into life-threatening conditions.

The CDC estimates an average of 700 deaths per year from heat-related causes, and about 1,300 per year from cold-related causes. Deaths from cold exposure and heat stroke are generally associated with outdoor activities, but in the event of a widespread disaster where air conditioning, fans, and heating systems may be inoperable, hypothermia and hyperthermia could be a major cause of death. Most of today's citizens are accustomed to heated and air-conditioned homes and vehicles, making them more vulnerable to prolonged exposure to excessive heat or cold.

Heat-Related Injuries
Even without access to air conditioning, heat-related injuries can be prevented. Limiting exercise, maintaining hydration, and taking frequent rests in the shade can help the body's cooling system. Be aware that heat exposure is cumulative over days, so these affects can develop quickly after several days of exposure. While people living in humid conditions are aware of sweating, those in dry desert-like environments may feel cool and dry because of evaporation but may be suddenly struck by the symptoms of dehydration and even heat stroke. Thirst is not a reliable indicator of hydration, so drink plenty of water in hot environments regardless of thirst, and be alert for the signs of heat exhaustion and heat stroke.

Heat Cramps

While heat cramps can be temporarily debilitating, they are not life threatening. Excessive exertion in a hot environment will generate copious sweating as the body works to keep the body core cool. This sweating can result in dehydration and loss of electrolytes from the muscle cells. This loss of water and electrolytes can result in cramping.

Treatment of Heat Cramps

1. Have the patient sit or lie down until the cramps subside.
2. Give the patient water and electrolyte solutions such as Gatorade™.
3. Get the patient into a cool environment and let them rest until the body rebalances the electrolytes in the muscles.
4. Evaluate the patient for the development of heat exhaustion or heat stroke

Heat Exhaustion

The most common illness resulting from exposure to high environmental temperatures is heat exhaustion. Profuse sweating is usually sufficient to cool the body, as long as the sweat is able to evaporate freely. If the person is wearing heavy clothing or the humidity is high, sweat is not able to evaporate and cool the body. Profuse sweating also depletes the body's water and electrolytes. Heat exhaustion is a form of mild hypovolemic shock.

Signs of Heat Exhaustion

1. Feeling weak, faint, or dizzy.
2. Cold, clammy skin.
3. Nausea or headache.
4. Rapid pulse.
5. Normal or slightly elevated temperature.

Treatment of Heat Exhaustion

1. Get the patient out of the sun and hot environment.
2. Get the patient to sit or lie down.
3. Remove any heavy or tight clothing.

4. If the patient is conscious and alert, provide plenty of water and/or electrolyte solutions such as Gatorade.
5. If the patient is not conscious and alert, do not attempt to force fluids.
6. The patient should begin to recover within about 30 minutes, but if the patient's level of consciousness continues to decline, more vigorous cooling efforts and immediate transportation to a medical facility is recommended.

HEAT STROKE

While heat cramps and heat exhaustion are easily treatable conditions, heat stroke is a true, life-threatening, medical emergency. Heat stroke results from prolonged exposure to high temperatures, where the body's regulatory mechanisms are overwhelmed and fail. If left untreated, heat stroke will always result in death. Heat stroke may develop if heat exhaustion is not treated effectively.

Signs of Heat Stroke

1. Red, dry skin is the primary indicator of heat stroke. The body's main method of cooling is sweating, and this system is failing.
2. Profound weakness.
3. A falling level of consciousness, leading to unconsciousness.
4. A rapidly rising body temperature.
5. Rapid pulse that weakens as the patient becomes unresponsive.
6. Falling blood pressure as the patient becomes unresponsive.

Treatment of Heat Stroke

1. Treatment must be initiated immediately. Waiting for an ambulance or transporting to a medical facility is secondary to immediate cooling of the patient.
2. Get the patient out of the hot environment and into an air-conditioned building or vehicle.
3. Cool the patient by any means available such as a cold water bath, cold wet towels, and cold packs under the arm pits, on both sides of the neck, and in the groin where blood circulation will cool the blood going to the core.
4. Transport to emergency care while continuing cooling efforts.

Cold-Related Injuries

Death from hypothermia usually occurs when the body's core temperature drops below 80 degrees. While often associated with exposure to subzero temperatures, hypothermia can develop from prolonged exposure to "chilly" conditions. If there is a golden rule of outdoor survival it should be "don't get wet." Wet or damp clothing loses most of its insulating value. Adequate nourishment is also important to the prevention of hypothermia. A marathon runner on a cool, 60-degree Fahrenheit day can develop hypothermia at the end of the race because he or she has (1) become soaked with sweat, and (2) used up all the internal metabolic energy reserves that otherwise could produce warmth. It is essential to understand that nature always strives to equalize temperature between you and the environment, so on 60-degree Fahrenheit day, the only thing keeping your body from being a deadly 60 degrees is your clothing and your body's metabolizing of food to generate heat energy.

PREVENTION OF HYPOTHERMIA

✚ Dress for what the weather could be, not what it is. Wearing shorts and a T-shirt on a mild day may be sufficient, but if you are unable to access shelter or caught in a sudden rainstorm, or the temperature drops suddenly, you could quickly develop hypothermia. Carrying a sweater, cap, and rain poncho is always advisable.

✚ Maintain adequate nourishment. Cold conditions require the body to burn more calories just to maintain the body's core temperature. Eating more high calorie foods when cold exposure is anticipated provides more fuel for your "internal furnace." Having energy bars in the pockets of cold weather clothing could be lifesaving.

✚ Always cover your head. The brain receives 20 percent of the body's blood supply, so the head can radiate a significant amount of heat. Wool caps are an essential part of all outdoor survival gear.

✚ Stay dry at all costs. Wearing wet clothing is equivalent to being in cold water. Always have a rain poncho on hand. Do not get wet trying to start a fire in the rain; seek the closest available shelter.

✚ Get out of the wind, as wind will carry away body heat through convection.

✚ When possible, cover the mouth and nose with a mask or scarf. Respiration is a major source of heat loss.

✚ Avoid prolonged contact with cold ground or other cold surfaces. These surfaces will suck heat from your body through conduction.

✚ Drink warm liquid in cold conditions. Warm drinks bring warmth to the body's core and essential organs. Never consume alcoholic beverages in cold conditions as they will accelerate cooling.

Signs of Hypothermia

1. When the body temperature drops below 97 degrees, shivering will develop as the body attempts to generate heat. Goosebumps develop and the patient is unable to perform complex manual tasks. These are early signs of impending hypothermia.

2. Intense shivering combined with poor muscle coordination, confusion, and a stumbling gait are the first indicators of developing hypothermia.

3. When shivering stops and the patient becomes incoherent or irrational and has difficulty speaking or walking, chronic hypothermia has developed. If action is not taken immediately, the patient will regress through the following conditions:

   ✚ Muscular rigidity, stupor, slowing respirations and pulse rate, and pupil dilation.

   ✚ Unconsciousness, erratic heartbeat and respiration, and loss of muscle reflex.

   ✚ Death. The lowest body core temperature survived by a patient was 64 degrees Fahrenheit, but most patients will expire with a core temperature between 75 and 80 degrees.

Once a person has developed signs of chronic hypothermia, just getting them into a warm room or vehicle will not halt the progression toward more severe cardiac and respiratory signs and death, because at this point the patient's metabolic "furnace" has shut down, and the patient will continue to cool to room temperature which is fatal. Ideally the patient should be warmed from the inside out in a medical facility. Unlike the treatment for hyperthermia, a hypothermic patient should not be rapidly rewarmed externally. The body will attempt to maintain the internal core temperature by reducing circulation from the extremities and skin, thus isolating cold blood in these areas. Rapid external warming will open these external blood vessels, pouring colder blood into the heart and vital organs, resulting in cardiac arrhythmias or fibrillation.

TREATMENT FOR HYPOTHERMIA

1. Move the patient to a warm room or vehicle.
2. Remove wet clothing from the patient and wrap them in warm dry blankets or a sleeping bag.
3. If the patient is fully conscious, provide warm, sweet liquids to drink.
4. Never provide alcoholic beverages as these will accelerate body cooling.
5. Never try to warm a chronic hypothermia patient by rubbing the arms, immersing arms in warm water, or placing warm packs, as this will release cold blood to the vital organs.
6. Monitor level of consciousness for signs of progressive conditions.
7. Maintain airway and administer CPR if necessary.
8. If immediate access to a hospital is not available and the patient has developed signs of hypothermia, place them into a sleeping bag or under heavy blankets with a person who is not experiencing hypothermia.
9. Even if a person is apparently dead in the cold, get them to professional care. The medical mantra for hypothermia is that "you are not dead until you are warm dead." Patients have been revived several hours after apparent death when the body was in the cold.

FROSTBITE

Frostbite is a serious localized injury resulting from the actual freezing of tissue. The severity of frostbite is dependent on how long the affected part is frozen and the depth of the damage. The consequences of frostbite can range from localized pain and swelling as circulation is restored to extensive loss of tissue, gangrene, and the necessity of amputation.

Signs of Frostbite

1. Early stages of frostbite are skin redness and being tender to the touch.
2. Hard and cold feeling to the skin.
3. White, yellow, or blue-white skin coloration.
4. Loss of sensation to touch.

Treatment of Frostbite

1. Remove any cold wet clothing that is covering the affected extremity.
2. Evaluate and treat the patient as needed for hypothermia.
3. The frostbitten part should be immersed in warm (100 to 112 degree) water until color and feeling returns.
4. Never thaw a frostbitten extremity if there is any danger of it being refrozen, as refreezing will do greater damage than leaving the part frozen.
5. Cover the affected part with a soft sterile dressing and get the patient to professional care as soon as possible.

IMMERSION FOOT

Also referred to as "trench foot," this results from extended exposure to cold, wet conditions, but actual freezing has not occurred. The condition is common among outdoor workers, hikers, and hunters who stand or walk in cold water for prolonged periods.

Signs of Immersion Foot

1. Feeling of coldness
2. Pale wrinkled tissue
3. Tingling sensation
4. Itching
5. Numbness
6. Pain when exposed to heat
7. Swelling
8. Occasional blistering

Treatment of Immersion Foot

1. Dry and clean the affected area.
2. Keep the foot or feet elevated.
3. Apply warm compresses for five minutes on, five minutes off.
4. Potassium permanganate foot baths may help to reduce swelling.
5. Be alert for the development of infection indicated by a foul odor, pus, spreading redness, and fever. If any of these signs develop seek medical attention immediately

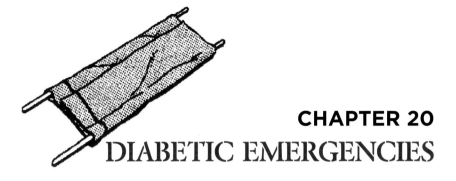

CHAPTER 20
DIABETIC EMERGENCIES

The CDC estimates that there are over 34 million diabetics in the United States, and of these, 8 to 10 million are undiagnosed. The disease is caused by the body's inability to metabolize sugar (glucose) because cells in the pancreas are unable to supply adequate insulin. Insulin enables glucose to enter the cell bodies. Sugar is as vital as oxygen to brain cells, and when it is sugar deprived, the brain will rapidly sustain permanent damage. When sugar cannot be used by the tissues, the levels of sugar in the blood will rise to extremely high levels. When sugar is not available as an energy source, the body metabolizes fat. Acids called ketones are produced when fat is used for energy in place of sugar. In uncontrolled diabetes, elevated levels of ketones can result in the development of diabetic ketoacidosis. Diabetic ketoacidosis causes stomach pain, vomiting, and deep rapid respirations. If the patient is not provided with fluids and insulin, the condition will progress into diabetic coma and death. Diabetics should monitor their blood sugar levels, manage their diet, and/or take insulin to regulate their glucose levels. When these measures are inadequate, the patient will experience a diabetic emergency.

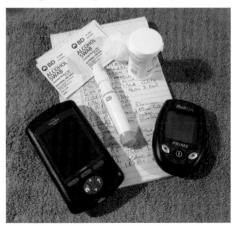

Diabetics should carry a kit that may include injectable insulin or devices to monitor and control their insulin pump. They usually track their food and insulin intake.

The two major medical emergencies resulting from poorly managed diabetes are diabetic coma and insulin shock. It can be difficult for the first aider to differentiate between the two conditions.

Diabetic Coma

Excessive sugar (glucose) in the blood does not in itself cause diabetic coma, but excessive waste in the blood and the loss of fluids causes problems.

✚ Diabetic coma can result from a patient taking insufficient insulin.

✚ The patient may have overeaten.

✚ The patient may be undergoing some stress or illness.

Ketoacidosis develops slowly over hours or even days and may result in the patient being found comatose.

Signs of Diabetic Coma

1. Rapid, deep sighing respirations
2. Sweet fruity breath odor, often mistaken for alcohol
3. Dry warm skin
4. Sunken eyes
5. Weak and rapid pulse
6. Normal or slightly low blood pressure
7. Deteriorated level of consciousness

Insulin Shock

As the name implies, insulin shock results from the patient taking too much insulin, and/or not eating enough food. The result is that there is too little blood sugar in the blood to supply the brain. Brain damage can occur if the blood sugar remains deficient. Insulin shock can develop very quickly.

Signs of Insulin Shock

1. Normal or rapid respiration
2. Pale moist skin (opposite of diabetic coma)
3. Profuse sweating
4. Headache and dizziness

5. Rapid pulse
6. Aggressiveness or unusual behavior
7. Marked hunger
8. Fainting, seizures, and coma

Diagnosis of a Diabetic Condition

In addition to the signs and symptoms listed above, the conscious patient can usually tell the first aider about their condition. Family members may also be able to provide information, and diabetics often have identifying necklaces, wristbands, or cards. Insulin-dependent diabetics usually carry injection kits and an insulin supply.

The following two questions should be asked of the patient: 1. Have you eaten today? 2. Have you taken your insulin today?

Treatment of Diabetic Coma and Insulin Shock

1. If the patient has eaten but not taken insulin, the problem is probably diabetic coma. Encourage the patient to take their insulin and get them to professional medical care.
2. If the patient has taken their insulin but has not eaten and is still conscious, provide sugar, soft drinks, orange juice, or other sweet liquids. If they are unconscious or semi-conscious, place glucose paste or sugar under the tongue. Once they recover full consciousness, encourage them to eat a candy bar or similar food. Even if the patient recovers, get them to medical care as soon as possible.
3. If in doubt, provide sugar, as this can do no harm even if the final diagnosis is diabetic coma.

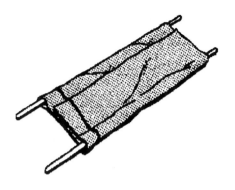

CHAPTER 21
STROKE

S trokes are usually associated with old-age, but they can afflict younger people as well. Recent studies indicate that physical and psychological trauma can increase a patient's likelihood of suffering a stroke. Those suffering from post-traumatic stress disorder (PTSD) have been found to have a higher incidence of stroke. PTSD can result from the stress created by natural disaster, combat, civil disorder, or the loss of a loved one, thus stroke is a potential disaster survival–related disorder. Violent trauma that may have caused a head injury or a brain injury that can generate hemorrhagic stroke days after the original incident. While there is little the first aider can do to prevent or treat stroke, early recognition and immediate access to professional care intervention are critically important. It has been found that stroke victims that get to the emergency room within one hour of onset have a much higher rate recovery than those whose care is delayed.

Causes of Stroke

Stroke or cerebrovascular accident (CVA) are usually caused by one of three events that interrupt the flow of blood to part of the brain.

Clotting of the cerebral arteries. This occurs from blockage of the arteries, usually caused by a buildup of cholesterol that narrows the passage inside the artery, promoting the formation of blood clots and complete blockage of blood flow. This is known as a thrombosis and is the most common cause of stroke.

Rupture of cerebral arteries. This problem can be caused by a congenital weakness in the artery or from hypertension. The rupture causes impaired circulation in the brain, while causing brain damage. These are referred to as aneurysms and are the most common cause of strokes in younger, healthier adults.

Obstruction of cerebral arteries. These strokes are caused by clots that form in other parts of the body and then travel to the cerebral arteries. They can also be caused by degenerating debris from the artery walls. Clot formation can result from severe injuries and illness. Gunshot wounds have been known to cause clots that break loose. There is some evidence that COVID-19 infections have generated clots that cause brain and heart complications.

The first aider should be alert for the signs of stroke in the elderly, anyone who has suffered trauma, and anyone who has contracted a long-term illness or severe soft-tissue injury.

Signs and Symptoms of Stroke

The signs and symptoms of a stroke are distinctive and unmistakable. They result from the interruption of blood supply or intercranial pressure to one side of the brain.

1. Sudden weakness, numbness, or paralysis of the extremities on one side (seldom both) of the body.
2. Sudden weakness and numbness on one side of the face.
3. Dimness in vision in one eye.
4. Difficulty swallowing, breathing, and speaking.
5. Diminished level of consciousness, from confusion to coma.
6. Sudden loss of balance, dizziness, or unexplained falls.
7. Sudden severe headache often followed by unconsciousness.

Stroke Victim Assessment

The acronym **FAST** is used to guide the first aider in recognition of a stroke.

+   **Face.** Ask the patient to smile. Observe for a noticeable face droop on one side of the mouth.
+   **Arms.** Ask the patient to hold both arms out straight to the side. Watch for one arm to sag downward.
+   **Speech.** Ask the patient to recite a simple phrase such as "Mary had a little lamb." Note slurred or muddled speech.
+   **Time.** If these signs are evident, do not waste further time. Get the patient to an ER!

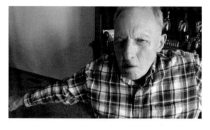

One-sided facial droop and arm downward drift are clear signs of a stroke.

Care of Stroke Victims

The ability to treat or reverse the causes of a stroke is far beyond the capabilities of first aiders. Supportive care and immediate access to a hospital is the only course of action available. Here are the only things you can do.

1. Call an ambulance or transport the patient to a hospital immediately upon recognition of the signs of a stroke!
2. Monitor and maintain the patient's airway and breathing.
3. Keep the patient warm and comfortable.
4. If transporting the patient yourself, do so in the approved, prone-on-disabled-side position.
5. Speak gently to the patient even if they seem to be unconscious, be aware that they may be able to hear you. Avoid negative remarks.

Positioning and Transport of Stroke Victims

When it is necessary for first aiders to transport an unconscious or semi-conscious stroke patient themselves, the patient should be positioned on a well-padded board or stretcher, with the disabled side down. This prevents them from swallowing or inhaling sputum and vomit, while freeing their still useful extremities.

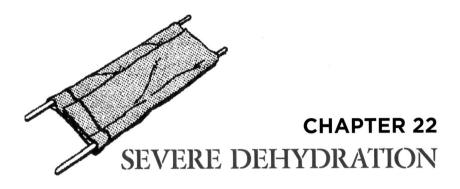

CHAPTER 22
SEVERE DEHYDRATION

One of the chief causes of death from more serious illnesses is dehydration. Most communicable diseases and radiation sickness cause sweating, vomiting, and diarrhea. In addition, many of these conditions also cause internal bleeding and sepsis. At the same time, the patient may not be able to intake fluids orally due to nausea or loss of consciousness. Deprived of fluids, the blood pressure drops, and the cells and organs begin to die. Critical electrolytes needed by the heart are not available, and death is inevitable unless fluids can be restored. This is why intravenous fluids are almost always provided to ill patients. Unfortunately, IV equipment and skills may not be available in the worst-case survival situations. In the event of massive epidemics or radiation exposure, the survivor may be forced to care for critically ill and dehydrated patients at home or in the field.

While maintaining hydration alone will not guarantee recovery, it certainly improves the patient's chances. When the patient can tolerate oral hydration, the following is recommended:

8 tsp. of sugar + 1 tsp. of salt to 1 liter of water. Provide small 4 oz. drinks every hour.

Caution: Giving water or other liquids to an unconscious, semiconscious, or seriously injured patient may cause them to vomit and aspirate.

Causes of Dehydration

1. Prolonged exposure to a hot, dry environment without drinking enough water.
2. Prolonged or chronic illness.
3. Sustained vomiting, diarrhea.
4. Profuse and sustained sweating and fever.
5. Severe and extensive burns.
6. Poor hydration habits. Low water intake.

Effects and Signs of Dehydration

Chronic dehydration is a common condition affecting a significant portion of the population and the cause of several unpleasant health conditions. Thirst is a poor indication of the need for hydration. Some of the effects and symptoms of dehydration are listed below.

1. Chronic dry eyes can be a sign of inadequate hydration.
2. Constipation is often caused by inadequate fluid in the digestive tract.
3. Brain fog and the inability to concentrate can often be traced to dehydration.
4. Sleeplessness can be caused by dehydration.
5. Abnormal irritability can be caused by dehydration.
6. Headaches are often caused by dehydration. The brain is actually drying up and separating from the inside of the skull. The classic "hangover" headache is the result of alcohol-caused dehydration. The water in coffee or taken with aspirin is usually more curative than the caffeine or pills.
7. Muscle cramps may be caused by inadequate fluids and electrolytes.
8. Cracked lips and dry cracked skin on the hands is an indication of dehydration.
9. Progressive dehydration will be indicated by a dry mouth, sunken eyes, and extreme thirst.
10. Yellow or even orange urine is a sure sign of dehydration.
11. Slow recovery of pinched tissue. Pinch the skin on the back of the patient's hand. It should rebound promptly. If it remains tented and slowly flattens, it is a reliable sign of poor hydration.
12. Thirst alone is not a reliable indicator of the need for hydration. The author experienced severe dehydration in the desert without being thirsty. IV fluids were required to reverse the effects.

Maintaining adequate hydration is essential to maintaining general health and provides you and your patients an advantage when injury or illness occurs. Hypovolemia and shock will set in faster if the patient is already dehydrated prior to the injury. The most common recommendation is for an adult to drink eight, eight-ounce glasses of water per day. If you drink a lot of coffee or consume lots of salty foods, you may need to drink more water to replace losses from urination. The potential for dehydration is particularly high for the following groups.

GROUPS SUSCEPTIBLE TO DEHYDRATION

1. Infants and young children, as they cannot verbalize their thirst and are more prone to diarrhea, vomiting, and fevers.
2. Elderly adults, who may not realize that they are thirsty and may have medical conditions that produce dehydration.
3. Individuals who are ill and may not want to drink or eat.
4. Diabetics may lose more water through frequent urination.
5. Those who are active outside in a hot environment and lose water through profuse sweating.
6. Those who are active for extended time in cold dry environment. Dry air (hot or cold) will suck moisture from the skin and respiration, and this can result in the unexpected onset of the effects of dehydration.

The bottom line is that it is easier to maintain hydration while the patient is healthy than it is to restore hydration to a sick patient who is possibly losing fluids through sweating, urination, diarrhea, and vomiting. Once the patient has lost full consciousness, oral fluids cannot be given, and the patient's condition will continue to decline unless intravenous fluids can be provided. The only other method for hydration of an unconscious patient is a technique known as proctoclysis.

Treatments for Dehydration

Once a patient has exhibited the signs of dehydration, action should be taken to provide water and electrolytes.

+ If the patient is vomiting frequently, over-the-counter medications such as Pepto Bismol, Kaopectate, or Milk of Magnesia can be given. Saltine crackers may be helpful in absorbing stomach acids while providing salt.
+ Patients who are losing fluid through frequent diarrhea can be hydrated and nourished with a solution of one teaspoon of salt and two tablespoons of sugar in one quart of water.

+ Conscious patients can be given small cups of the above hydration solution, and/or Gatorade, commercial electrolyte drinks, chicken broth, or tomato juice.
+ If the patient is unconscious or cannot tolerate oral fluids they should be taken to a facility where intravenous fluids (0.9% normal saline, lactated ringers, or dextrose 5% in water) can be administered.

PROCTOCLYSIS

When IV fluid administration is not available, proctoclysis is a practical alternative. The function of the large intestines and colon is to absorb water from the waste product. This water generally comes from the top end of the digestive system, but water injected into the other end will be absorbed just as effectively. Up until the 1930s, proctoclysis was widely utilized for fluid administration. Although not as effective as an IV, this method is safer for the untrained medic. IV administration can result in injuries, infections, and other complications whereas the colon is already designed to filter out unwanted materials.

While sterile water would be preferable, any clean water should be usable. Saline solution (9%) or electrolyte solutions could also be beneficial. Enema sets can usually be purchased for a few dollars at a pharmacy, or the improvised setups shown below can be assembled

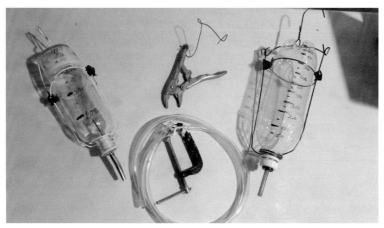

Improvised protoclysis system. The clamp taped to the tubing serves as a flow control. The calibrated bottles are wired so they can be hung above the patient while administering fluid into the rectum.

from available soft, 3/8-inch-diameter plastic tubing, bottles, wire, and clamps.

The patient should be positioned on their side. The tubing then must be coated with water-soluble gel and inserted gently about 10 inches into the rectum. The filled bottle or bag of fluid should be hung at least two feet above the patient. Flow rate is then controlled by the clamp device pinching the tubing. Slowly open the clamp to increase the flow. Excessive fluid discharge from the rectum will indicate too much flow. The bottles shown are calibrated in 50 and 100 cc increments. Experimentation will establish the effective rate for each patient.

Note the small holes drilled in the first three inches of the tubing. This will facilitate good fluid distribution if the end of the tubing is blocked by feces. It is also important to burn or smooth the tube end to avoid tearing the rectal tissue.

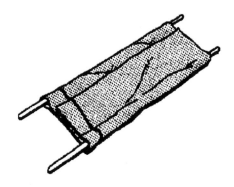

CHAPTER 23
POISONING

A poison can be any substance that, when swallowed, inhaled, or absorbed through the skin or mucus membranes, in even small amounts, can alter normal metabolism and/or damage or destroy cells. While most poisoning incidents in the United States result from drugs, a significant number of fatalities each year are the result of carbon monoxide, household chemicals, and contaminated food.

Carbon Monoxide Poisoning

Carbon monoxide is a deadly poison created by inefficient burning. This poison is particular dangerous because it is odorless and tasteless and can overcome victims without their being aware of its presence. Carbon monoxide replaces the oxygen in the red blood cells, making it impossible for oxygen to reach them. This results in serious damage to the tissues and death.

Common causes of carbon monoxide generation include the following:

1. Faulty heating systems or water heaters.
2. Obstructed heating vents or fireplace flues.
3. Burning of charcoal in an enclosed space.
4. Operation of kerosene or other heaters inside without adequate ventilation.
5. Running of internal combustion engines for vehicles or generators inside of an enclosed space.
6. As a component of smoke in a burning building.

During emergencies and disasters, the use of generators and unsafe heating systems makes the potential for carbon monoxide poisoning much more acute. Whole families and whole groups have been killed by carbon monoxide poisoning under such circumstances. While carbon monoxide alarms are a must for all homes, they are not to be regarded as one hundred percent reliable. If the signs and symptoms are there, act on them.

SIGN AND SYMPTOMS OF CARBON MONOXIDE POISONING

✚ Persistent mild headaches and sleepiness that affect everyone in the same house or building and seem to clear up when they go outdoors is a probable indication of developing carbon monoxide poisoning. The building should be evacuated and not reentered until checked by a professional or the fire department.

✚ Severe headache, weakness, nausea, vomiting, blurry vision, sleepiness, confusion, and breathing difficulty are signs of serious carbon monoxide poisoning. All victims must evacuate the building immediately. Call 911 to get immediate medical attention.

✚ Mild breathing difficulties may be the only sign that develops prior to sudden respiratory arrest.

✚ If carbon monoxide poisoning is suspected, the first aider must get the victim and all other occupants out of the building immediately, regardless of whether anyone else is exhibiting symptoms.

✚ While oxygen may be sufficient to revive victims of mild carbon monoxide exposure, severe cases often need to be placed in a hyperbaric chamber to flush the poison from the body.

Chemical Poisoning

Chemical poisoning can be the result of accidental ingestion of household chemicals or an accidental chemical release from a nearby factory, or it can be the result of a deliberate terrorist act. Our home and community environment is filled with hazardous and deadly chemical substances that can be accidentally or deliberately released. Releases can be the secondary result of other disasters such as floods, earthquakes, or fires. Civil disorder and terrorist activity can result in the intentional release of toxic chemical into the air and water supply of major population areas. In 2020, hackers attempted to increase the levels of chlorine in a town's water supply, and hackers could cause contamination to water supplies and catastrophic failures of safety systems for chemical processing facilities at any time.

The failure of safety systems at the Union Carbide insecticide production facility in Bhopal, India, in 1976 released methyl isocyanate gas that killed 3,787 people initially and another 25,000 later. In 1995, a terrorist group released Sarin gas into the Tokyo subway system, killing 13 and injuring 5,500. These examples illustrate the need for the first aider to be able recognize and respond to chemical exposure incidents.

COMMON HOUSEHOLD CHEMICAL POISONS

Antifreeze, insecticides, weed killer, cleaners, fungicides, paint thinner, ant poison, drain cleaner, bleach, ammonia, and hundreds of other common household products can be poisonous if ingested. The hazards, symptoms, and first aid recommendations are usually listed on the label. Never transfer chemicals to unlabeled containers. Follow the label directions for use. Keep chemicals and medications out of the reach of children.

If ingestion is suspected, call the Poison Control Hotline at 1-800-222-1222.

FIRST AID FOR CHEMICAL POISONING

1. Follow the instructions of the container label and/or those provided by poison control.
2. Water or milk may be given if the patient is experiencing gastric distress and irritation.
3. If instructed, induce vomiting by oral administration of three (two for children) teaspoons of syrup of ipecac followed by two glasses of water. The patient will vomit within 15 to 20 minutes.
4. Make sure the patient's airway is kept clear and that they do not aspirate vomited material.
5. Never induce vomiting if the poison is a corrosive such as acid or lye.
6. Never induce vomiting if there are obvious burns in the mouth or lips caused by the chemical.
7. Never induce vomiting if the patient is having convulsions or is not fully conscious.
8. Never induce vomiting if the patient has swallowed gasoline, bleach, lighter fluid, or other similar chemicals.

9. If instructed, a mixture of one tablespoon of activated charcoal in one eight-ounce glass of water may be given to absorb poison. Do not administer charcoal after syrup of ipecac as it will inhibit the action of the medication.

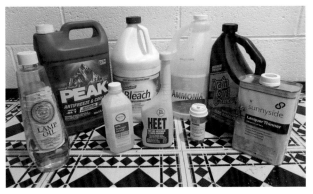

Common household poisons. Household ammonia and bleach generate chlorine gas when mixed. Spilled antifreeze often kills children and pets as it has a sweet taste. Prescription medications should be kept out of the reach of children and disposed of safely when no longer needed. Most pharmacies will take back unused pills for disposal.

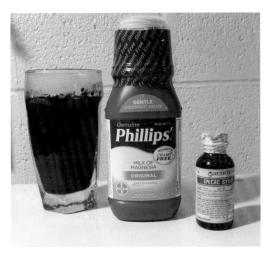

Poison treatments include activated charcoal to absorb the poison, Milk of Magnesia to dilute the poison and coat the stomach, and syrup of ipecac to induce vomiting. Treatment depends on the type of poison, label instructions, and guidance from poison control.

Terrorist Chemical Attacks

The manufacture and release of Sarin, a complex military poison, by a militant Japanese terrorist group in 1995 illustrates how easy it is for amateur chemists to create quantities of chemical warfare agents. Chlorine, ammonia, hydrogen cyanide, and other deadly chemicals are easily purchased or stolen. Toxins such as ricin and anthrax can be manufactured in any kitchen.

Chlorine is the major component of household bleach. Much stronger concentrations are used in industrial applications. Chlorine gas was used as a weapon during World War I. Its ubiquity makes it a likely candidate for terrorist actions and accidental releases. When even the mild (8.25%) household bleach solution is mixed with commercial ammonium hydroxide, chlorine gas is released. Accidental and deliberate combining of these two common chemicals has resulted in numerous respiratory injuries.

Chlorine gas is heavier than air and can concentrate in low areas and basements. Exposure results in severe respiratory irritation and breathing difficulty. Skin contact causes chemical burns. Eye contact will cause eye damage. Get an exposed patient to fresh air, remove contaminated clothing, and flush contaminated skin. Administer oxygen if available and call 911.

Ammonia and anhydrous ammonia are commonly used in industry and agriculture. The odor of ammonia is an excellent "warning property" and will usually force people to evacuate to fresh air well before permanent harm is done. If a victim is trapped or becomes unconscious within a high concentration of ammonia, death will result. Skin contact will cause chemical burns. Eye contact will cause eye damage. Responders should not attempt rescue without full skin, eye, and respiratory protection. Get an exposed patient to fresh air, remove contaminated clothing, and flush contaminated skin. Administer oxygen if available and call 911.

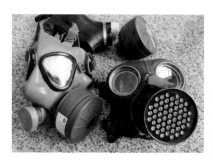

Gas masks such as these are seldom needed unless you live near to a chemical facility.

Hydrogen cyanide compounds and solutions are used in industry and have been used as chemical warfare agents. Accidental releases are particularly deadly. These chemicals are also transported by truck and rail through populated areas. Inhalation, skin contact, or ingestion can cause severe injury and death. Responders should not attempt rescue without full skin, eye, and respiratory protection. Get patient to fresh air, remove contaminated clothing, and flush contaminated skin. Administer oxygen if available and call 911.

Other Poisonous Chemicals

Chlorine, ammonia, and hydrogen cyanide are just three of the most common deadly chemicals that can be deliberately or accidental released into populated areas. The best source of information on these hazards is the *Emergency Response Guidebook*. Published every four years by the US Department of Transportation and available as a free, downloadable PDF or from J. J. Keller & Associates, Inc.

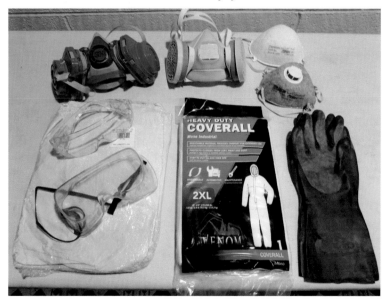

Respirators (top left) need to have specific filters for anticipated chemicals. The N95 dust/mist respirators are not intended for long-term exposure but are more easily kept available. Chemical protective suits, rubber gloves, and chemical goggles are required for exposure to corrosive substances. All of these products are available at industrial supply outlets and online.

at www.jjkeller.com. The book consists of five sets of color-coded pages that you can use to look up the chemical name or code number and be referred to appropriate response guide quickly. White pages provide general guidance and safety precautions. Yellow pages list chemicals by their ID numbers as they appear on all transport and storage containers, and the blue pages list chemical names in alphabetical order. The orange pages consist of response guides including health effects, first aid, protective equipment, and other hazards. Green pages show evacuation or shelter-in-place distances. There is also full information on how to read the label/signage on chemical trucks, railcars, and storage tanks. These books are standard carries on every ambulance and fire truck and are a good addition to any disaster response library or vehicle.

Bioterrorism Agents

Ricin is a potent toxin made from castor beans. The recipe for making ricin is available on the internet. Ricin-contaminated letters have been sent to government officials and others over the past ten years. Ricin can be aerosolized over a large area or group of people. Symptoms usually appear within few hours of exposure and death can occur within 36 to 72 hours. Symptoms include fever, vomiting, severe cough, abdominal pain, diarrhea, dehydration, and death. Exposure to a powdery substance and onset of symptoms by everyone exposed is an indicator of ricin poisoning. While the poisoning itself is not communicable, the victim may be contaminated and expose the first aider. Decontamination of the victim and full personal protection measures must be followed.

Anthrax is technically a biological agent rather than a chemical agent. It is one of the most likely agents to be used by bioterrorist, because it can be easily produced, it lasts a long time, and anthrax powder can be dispersed into air, or onto food and water easily. Anthrax spores are so small that they cannot usually be seen, tasted, or smelled. Like ricin, the powder has been used on mail. In one such incident, twenty-two people were infected and five died. Anthrax spores can be inhaled, injected, or absorbed through the skin. If deliberately spread, a victim could touch, inhale, and swallow the spores simultaneously.

✚ **Contact** exposure alone is the least dangerous anthrax exposure. The symptoms include raised, itchy bumps, swollen and sore lymph nodes, and flu-like symptoms.

✚ **Ingestion** of anthrax spores creates nausea, vomiting, bloody diarrhea, difficulty swallowing, abdominal pain, fever, and a swollen neck.

✚ **Inhalation** of anthrax spores initiates the most severe and deadly symptoms including flu-like symptoms, chest discomfort, nausea, coughing up blood, fever, painful swallowing, difficulty breathing, shock, and meningitis. As with ricin, decontamination of the victim and full personal protection measures must be followed.

Food Poisoning

Under emergency conditions, refrigeration may fail and available food may be contaminated. Terrorists have been known to intentionally contaminate food supplies. If some of the food supplies are deliberately contaminated, all foods may be suspect or even declared unsafe. This is another reason why one should always have at least six months of safe canned and dried foods at home.

Common Food Poisoning Sources

Toxin	Potential Source	Symptoms Onset
Salmonella	Raw meat, poultry, milk, eggs	1–3 days
Listeria	Processed meat, cheese, hotdogs, unpasteurized milk	9–48 hours
Rotavirus	Raw food products, contaminated water	1–3 days
Hepatitis A	Raw food products, contaminated water	28 days
Campylobacter	Meat, poultry, unpasteurized milk, contaminated water	2–5 days
Clostridium perfringens	Meat, stews, when kept at warm but not hot temperatures	8–16 hours
Giardia lamblia	Raw food products, contaminated water	1–2 weeks
Norovirus	Raw food products, contaminated water, shellfish	12–28 hours
Clostridium botulinum	Improperly canned foods, smoked fish, potatoes baked in aluminum foil, food kept warm for too long	12–72 hours

Toxin	Potential Source	Symptoms Onset
Staphylococcus aureus	Meat, vegetables, pastries, sauces, hand contact, coughing, sneezing	1–6 hours
Escherichia coli	Undercooked beef, unpasteurized milk, apple cider, contaminated water	1–8 days
Shigella	Raw seafood	24–48 hours
Vibrio vulnificus	Raw oysters, scallops, etc.; contaminated water	1–7 days

It should be obvious from the above table that under emergency conditions, all foods should be well cooked to an internal a temperature of 165 degrees Fahrenheit, and all water should be boiled for at least one minute or treated with 16 drops of bleach per gallon of water.

MILD FOOD POISONING SIGNS

1. Nausea and vomiting
2. Bloody diarrhea
3. Abdominal pain
4. Fever

SEVERE FOOD POISONING SIGNS

If these sign and symptoms are exhibited seek professional medical attention.

1. Extreme abdominal pain
2. Frequent vomiting
3. Inability to keep food down
4. Bloody vomit or diarrhea
5. Fever in excess of 102 degrees Fahrenheit
6. Weakness, blurred vision, and tingling in the arms

TREATMENT OF FOOD POISONING

1. Most food poisoning can be treated at home.
2. Administer over the counter medications such as Pepto-Bismol, Imodium, or Milk of Magnesia to control nausea, vomiting, and diarrhea.

3. Maintain the patient's hydration with electrolyte-enhanced sports drinks.

4. Avoid providing caffeinated beverages. Provide chamomile or peppermint tea instead.

5. Provide foods such as broth, rice, bananas, toast, saltine crackers, oatmeal, and jello to maintain strength.

6. Provide rest and monitor temperature.

Ingested Plant Poisoning

Many household and wild plants are poisonous if ingested. Wild poisonous plants include water hemlock, poke berries, oleander, white hellebore, deadly nightshade, and toadstool mushrooms. Children are the most often victims after nibbling on plant leaves. Plant poisoning can affect the circulatory system, nervous system, and gastrointestinal tract. Symptoms usually occur within 30 minutes of ingestion and can include the following:

1. Falling blood pressure
2. Rapid heart rate
3. Profuse sweating
4. Weakness
5. Cold moist clammy skin
6. Vomiting
7. Diarrhea
8. Intestinal cramps

There is no effective antidote for plant poisoning. Vomiting should be induced by administration of syrup of ipecac. The patient should be treated as for shock, but be alert to turn the patient to the recovery (side) position to prevent aspiration of vomit. Seek prompt professional medical attention.

Contact Plant Poisoning

Poison ivy, poison oak, and poison sumac are common sources of contact poisoning. After direct contact, the sap from the plants will cause skin irritation. If not washed off with soap and water, blisters may develop. Severe cases may require medical attention. Calamine lotion, baking soda, and colloidal oatmeal are common topical treatments for itching and oozing sores.

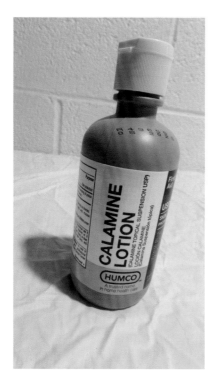

Calamine lotion is one of the most effective treatments for skin contact poisons. Wearing long sleeves and long pants when moving through plant growth is the best way to avoid this problem.

Note: Poisonous plants including oleander, poison ivy, poison oak, and poison sumac can produce poisonous smoke and vapors when burned. These vapors can generate severe respiratory, eye, and nervous system injury. Avoid burning these plants and smoke from brush fires that may include these plants.

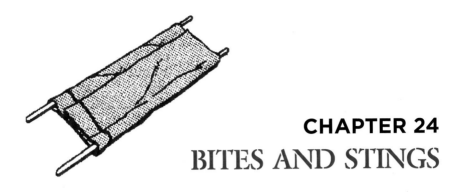

CHAPTER 24
BITES AND STINGS

A nimal bites, snake bites, and insect stings can develop into major health emergencies when they occur in the outdoors far from access to hospitals. In disaster situations, disease-carrying animals and insects could become a major health and safety concern. In addition to the bite injury, bites and stings can be the vectors for infectious diseases. If not treated promptly all animal bites and many insect stings can develop into serious infections.

Rat, Bat, and Wild Animal Bites

Rats are a common problem in many urban areas. After a disaster or unrest, rats may multiply and spread into the surrounding regions, spreading diseases and creating a hazard for residents. Rats were the primary carriers of the bubonic plague that killed 25 million people from 1348 to 1350 AD. Rats carry a variety of pathogens that can be spread through their bites, their fleas, or just their contact with the environment. Rats also carry rabies. Rabies is an always fatal disease of the brain that can only be prevented by immediate vaccination after the bite. If the patient has been bitten or scratched by a rat, bat, wild animal, or unvaccinated dog or cat they must be taken to a hospital immediately. If the animal can be killed or captured for examination, it may save the patient the necessity of these painful spinal injections. Tetanus is also associated with animal bites, and the first aider should get a tetanus booster shot every ten years.

Rate bite fever (spirillum) can be contracted from a rat bite, contact, or just being in a rat-infested environment. Symptoms of rat bite fever include fever, vomiting, headache, muscle and joint pain, swollen lymph nodes, swelling at the bite site, and a rash. Untreated rat bite fever can develop into complications involving the lungs, heart, kidneys, and brain. Respiratory protection should be used whenever rendering aid where rats may be present.

TREATMENT FOR ANIMAL BITES

1. Stop severe bleeding.
2. Thoroughly clean and flush the wound.
3. Apply an antiseptic ointment such as Triple Antibiotic or Neosporin™.
4. Cover the wound with a sterile bandage.
5. Check the wound frequently for signs of infection, including redness, swelling, heat, and pus.
6. Access professional medical attention promptly.
7. Assess the need for rabies vaccination and/or tetanus booster shots.

Effective antibiotics for animal bite infections include penicillin, amoxicillin, doxycycline, and erythromycins.

Insect Stings

Insect stings can lead to more serious complications including infection and anaphylactic shock. More people die each year from insect stings than from snake bites. The most common stinging insects are bees, wasps, hornets, and fire ants.

The symptoms of insect bites are:

1. Sudden pain
2. Swelling and redness
3. Heat
4. Itching
5. In some cases, a firm, whitish elevation of the skin

Bee stingers remain in the skin and inject venom for several minutes after the sting. Do not use tweezers to remove the stinger, as this will squeeze more venom into the wound. Scrape the stinger away with a knife edge. Patients with a history of allergic reactions to insect stings may carry injectable epinephrine and/or antihistamines.

Brown Recluse Spider Bites

Brown recluse spiders are dull brown in color and have a black violin shaped mark on their backs. They tend to live in wood piles and under rocks. The bite produces localized but severe tissue damage and a large, slow-healing ulcer in the skin. The bite becomes

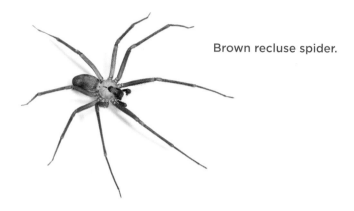

Brown recluse spider.

painful within a few hours. A red, swollen, and tender sore with a pale mottled center develops. A large scab of dead skin will develop into a deep ulcer.

There is no antivenom for this bite. Treatment must be focused on prevention of infection with antibiotics. Serious infections and even the development of necrotizing fasciitis (flesh-eating disease) may result.

Signs of infection and/or necrotizing fasciitis include the following:

+ Redness and swelling around the bite
+ Redness radiating from the bite area
+ Hardening of the skin and a shiny, dead appearance
+ Signs of gangrene

Infections can be treated with the same antibiotics as for other bites, but necrotizing fasciitis must be treated in the hospital with massive amounts of intravenous antibiotics to avoid amputations or death.

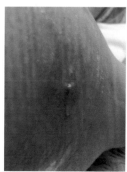

Brown recluse spider bite that became infected and required antibiotics.

Black Widow Spider Bites

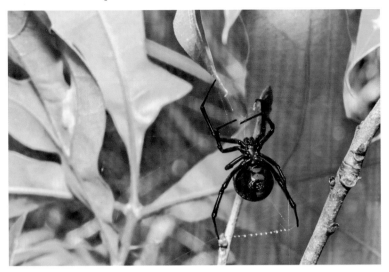

Black widow spider.

The black widow spider is approximately one inch long, black with a distinctive red or orange hourglass marking. The venom is a neurotoxin that attacks the spinal nerves of those bitten. The victim may not feel the initial bite but will develop symptoms over 24 hours. The symptoms include the following:

1. Severe cramps
2. Rigidity of the abdomen
3. Tightness of the chest
4. Difficulty breathing
5. Dizziness
6. Sweating
7. Nausea and vomiting
8. Skin rash

Symptoms can be severe but are rarely fatal, and usually subside within 24 hours. Antivenin is available but is seldom required except when the patient is a child.

Scorpion Stings

The symptoms of most scorpion stings include localized swelling, pain, and discoloration, but the Arizona scorpion's venom can produce a severe reaction that includes muscle contractions, excessive salivation, convulsions, hypertension, and cardiac failure. Those bitten by suspected Arizona scorpions must be rushed to an emergency room as soon as possible. The first aider should be prepared to administer CPR and use an AED if available. The Arizona scorpion resides only in Arizona, and an antivenin is available.

Tick Bites

Ticks carry diseases including Rocky Mountain spotted fever and Lyme disease. When in tick-infested areas, check the whole body for ticks daily. To remove ticks:

1. Grasp the tick with pointed tweezers as close to the skin as possible.
2. Pull evenly and slowly, without twisting.
3. Alternative: Apply alcohol to make the tick back out of the wound.
4. Clean the bite site with alcohol or soap and water.
5. Consult healthcare provider if Lyme disease is prevalent in the area.
6. Watch for the development of the following symptoms of Lyme disease:
   + Rash
   + Fever
   + Fatigue
   + Headache
   + Swelling of extremities and neck
   + Muscle pain
   + Swollen joints

The development of any of these symptoms should generate immediate transport to professional care. The preferred antibiotic for Lyme disease is doxycycline. In severe cases, Lyme disease can lead to arthritis, cardiac and neurological disorders, and death.

Snake Bites

Some 80,000 people per year worldwide die of venomous snake bites, but very few of these deaths occur in the United States. Under emergency conditions where large numbers of people might be forced to travel through or camp in wilderness locations, snake bite incidents could increase significantly. There are two types of venomous snakes in the United States.

Pit Vipers, including rattlesnakes, cottonmouths, copperheads, and water moccasins, are identifiable by their triangular flat heads, and a pit just behind the nostrils. They inject venom by striking with their two fangs. The venom is a tissue destroyer, intended to begin the digestive process of typical prey such as rabbits and prairie dogs. In humans, it kills tissue around the bite and spreads outward. In addition to two fang marks, sign of envenomation will start with burning pain at the site. The venom destroys tissue and interferes with blood clotting, resulting in spreading and painful bruising. Systemic symptoms may include sweating, weakness, fainting, and shock.

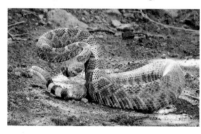

A rattlesnake preparing to strike.

Coral Snakes are members of the cobra family and do not have fangs. Coral snakes are shy and will usually avoid biting. They have teeth and need to chew the venom into the victim, leaving a horseshoe-shaped wound. They cannot open their mouth and strike like a pit viper, so they tend to bite fingers, toes, feet, and hands rather than larger surfaces. They are usually found in Florida and in the desert, and are easily identified by adjoining red and yellow rings around their bodies.

The old rhyme goes: "Red and yellow kill a fellow; red and black venom lack." Coral snake venom is a powerful neurotoxin that affects the victim's nervous system within a few hours. Symptoms of coral snake envenomation include strange behavior, increasing paralysis of eye movements, and increasing respiratory paralysis.

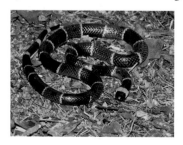

Coral snake with the distinctive red band bracketed by yellow bands.

TREATMENT FOR SNAKE BITE

Snake bite treatments are controversial and change frequently. Early treatment involved making small incisions at the wound site and applying suction to draw out the venom, but it was found that the venom had already circulated within minutes of the strike and the cuts only worsened the injury. More recently, the application of ice to the wounded extremity was recommended to slow the spread of the venom, but this has now been discounted as ineffective and damaging. The actions below are the generally accepted procedures pending access to antivenin.

1. Keep the patient calm and immobile, as agitation will speed the spread of the venom.
2. Clean the wound site with soap and water or mild antiseptic.
3. Wrap soft rubber tubing above and below the injury site to reduce peripheral circulation of the venom, but do not apply a tourniquet.
4. Splint the affected extremity to reduce movement.
5. Elevation of the affected limb may slow the spread of venom.
6. If you can kill the snake and bring it to the hospital, it will help medical providers select the correct antivenin.
7. Monitor vital signs and treat for shock if appropriate.
8. Transport the patient to the nearest medical facility
9. Be aware that about one-third of all snake bites are not envenomed but can still cause infection. Therefore, cleaning the wound and the application of antibiotic ointment is always appropriate.

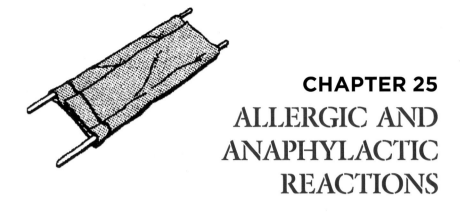

CHAPTER 25
ALLERGIC AND ANAPHYLACTIC REACTIONS

The first aider should be alert for the development of allergic reactions to a variety of substances. Different allergens can affect different tissues in the body in different ways. For example:

1. Effects on the nose and throat include sneezing, stuffiness, runny nose, and itching of the throat and eyes.
2. Effects on the skin include hives, flushing, and rash.
3. Effects on the bronchial tissue include swelling, wheezing, coughing, and difficulty breathing. These are especially dangerous anaphylactic signs that require immediate action.
4. Effects on the intestinal tract include nausea, vomiting, abdominal pain, cramps, and diarrhea.
5. In some cases, an allergic reaction can affect the brain, causing headaches.

Common Allergens

Allergens can enter the body through inhalation, skin contact, injection, or ingestion. Some of the most common sources of allergic reactions include the following:

Inhaled Allergens

+   Mold spores
+   Pollen
+   Animal dander
+   Dust mites
+   Cockroaches

Contact Allergens

+ Latex, including latex gloves
+ Some fabrics
+ Some insecticides
+ Some industrial chemicals
+ Plants such as poison oak, poison sumac, and poison ivy

Ingested Allergens

+ Nuts and legumes, including peanuts and peanut butter
+ Strawberries
+ Carrots
+ Wheat and grain products

Individuals with food allergies often carry prescription antihistamines or epinephrine injectors.

Injected Allergens: Bee, wasp, and hornet stings are the most common source of an allergic reaction and can quickly progress to full-blown anaphylaxis if epinephrine is not administered.

Drug Allergens

The first aider must be especially alert for those who may be allergic to medications. Under emergency conditions, it may be necessary to administer various medications and antibiotics without access to professional medical care. Be sure to ask the patient about any known allergies before administering any medication and be alert for signs of an allergic reaction. Medications that some individuals are allergic to include the following:

+ Aspirin
+ Sulfa drugs
+ Amoxicillin
+ Ampicillin
+ Penicillin
+ Tetracycline
+ Ibuprofen
+ Naproxen
+ Insulin

Anaphylactic Shock

Anaphylactic shock is a severe allergic reaction that often results in death unless promptly reversed. Anaphylaxis is more often developed from a reaction to drugs, foods, and stings, but it can develop from contact and inhaled allergens as well. Signs of developing anaphylaxis include the following:

✚ Difficulty breathing.
✚ Becoming hoarse.
✚ Wheezing respirations are a sign that the trachea is closing up.
✚ Swelling around the face, mouth, eyes, hands, and feet.
✚ Stomach cramps, nausea, and vomiting.
✚ Dizziness and loss of consciousness.

These extreme signs of anaphylaxis will usually lead to death unless epinephrine is administered promptly.

Antihistamines and Epinephrine

Antihistamines block the histamine receptors in the airway, blood vessels, stomach, and esophagus. These receptors are stimulated by allergens that cause inflammation of the tissues and narrowing of the airway. Antihistamines are often carried by those suffering from common allergies such as hay fever and are effective against mild allergic reactions but are not sufficient to revers anaphylaxis. Antihistamines should be included in every first aid kit. When no access to epinephrine is available, antihistamines may be the only alternative in managing anaphylactic shock. Common antihistamines include Allegra (fexofenadine), Aller-Tec (cetirizine), Benadryl (diphenhydramine), and Clarinex (desloratadine).

Epinephrine is the preferred drug for managing anaphylaxis. Epinephrine autoinjectors are commonly carried by people who have known allergies. Autoinjectors deliver 0.3 mg doses of epinephrine. The injection is delivered intramuscular, to the outer side of the thigh. In severe cases, a second dose may be required. Minor side effects of epinephrine include anxiety, headache, tremors, and palpitations. While epinephrine loses some effectiveness over time and expires after 12 to 18 months, it is better to use an expired device than not to use it in an emergency situation.

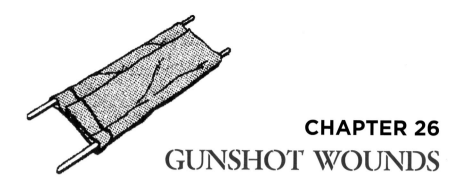

CHAPTER 26
GUNSHOT WOUNDS

The potential for the first aider encountering a gunshot wound victim increase as violent crime and civil unrest become more prevalent. Any type of large-scale disaster situation will inevitably generate violence. While those preparing to survive such events may choose to arm themselves for self and family defense, it must be assumed that if you may need to shoot, you have the potential of being shot. Therefore acquiring the skills and equipment to survive gunshot wounds must be as important as acquiring weapons and shooting skills.

Scene Safety

Scene safety is THE most important element of responding to a bullet wound incident. EMS first responders will usually not even enter a gunshot scene until police have secured the area. A first aider responding to the needs of a family member or neighbor may have the imperative to act regardless of risk. The tendency to develop tunnel vision and not notice that the shooter or shooters are still around or may return must be overcome. Observe the entire area. Do not assume that witnesses are not, in fact, the shooters. Consider if this was a close contact or a sniper-caused event. Be sure that no firearms are lying around. If so, secure or disassemble them before continuing. Consider the possibility that the victim may also be a shooter and may have a concealed weapon. If you train for first aid with a family or group, have an armed security person or persons covering you as you render first aid. This is one of the cases where moving a victim to a secure, covered (bullet-proof) location before rendering further aid is justifiable.

Gunshot Effects

The effects of a gunshot wound are dependent on velocity of the bullet, the type of bullet, the part of the body shot, and the route of the bullet once it enters the body.

Velocity

Bullet velocities are classified as low velocity when the muzzle velocity is less than 2,000 feet per second. These are usual handgun rounds such as .22, .380, .38, .40, and .45 caliber and 9-millimeter. These rounds produce less internal tissue damage and less penetration. High velocity rounds travel at speeds from 2,200 feet per second to over 4,000 feet per second. The shockwave from high-velocity bullets destroys tissue adjoining the primary wound track, creating a deep and large area of dead tissue with the potential for infection and gangrene. Of course, the muzzle velocity decreases with the distance from the muzzle to the target.

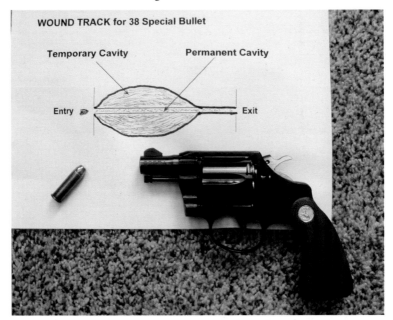

This low-velocity .38 Special bullet makes only a narrow permanent cavity. The temporary cavity only exists during impact.

Type of Bullet

The type of ammunition that created the wound greatly impacts the type of wound created. For example: .22 long rifle rounds are relatively small and low velocity but can ricochet around inside the body. In one case a .22 LR round entered the left-front shoulder, ricocheted off the scapula, and penetrated the heart, aorta, and lung, before coming to rest near the right hip. Hollow-point bullets expand and make large exit wounds. Defense rounds are designed to expend their energy in stopping an assailant by fragmenting inside the body. The hard nose of armor-piercing ammunition will go cleanly through the body. The 7.62-mm bullets from AK-47 rifles are notorious for tumbling through the body, creating a massive wound track and exiting out of line with the entry wound.

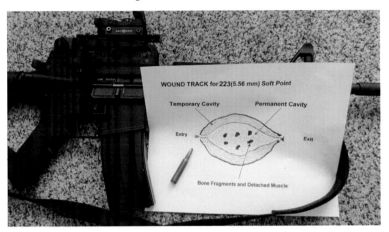

The .223 caliber, high-velocity round from an AR-15 causes a massive permanent cavity of dead or damaged tissue and leaves fragments in the cavity, with a high probability of major blood loss, shock, and infection.

POINT OF ENTRY

Where the bullet enters has important implications regarding the potential damage to and the survival of the victim. Bullets that penetrate the skull are almost always fatal, but some have been survived. Bullets into or through the thorax can strike the heart or major blood vessels, causing immediate death, but rounds that only penetrate the relatively hollow lung tissue are often survivable and can be treated as hemothorax and pneumothorax. Abdominal gunshot wounds are particularly serious, as they inevitably involve the solid organs and intestines. While they are seldom immediately fatal, only prompt surgical intervention can save these victims. Military data indicates that from 60 to 70 percent of combat bullet wounds were to the arms and legs. Gunshot wounds to the extremities are usually survivable if prompt action is taken to stop arterial bleeding and shock.

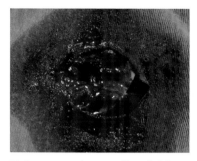
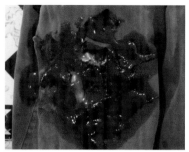

Entry wounds are often fairly small.

Exit wounds can be quite spectacular.

BULLET TRAJECTORY

A bullet may enter from high, low, or the side and continue upward, downward, or across through the body. Generally, the position of the victim, the direction from which the gun was fired, and the line between the entry and exit wounds should indicate what organs may have been impacted. The potential for bullet tumbling or ricochet must always be considered.

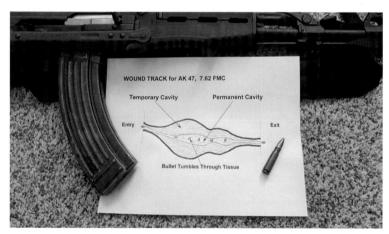

High-velocity rounds from AK-47 and AKM rifles tend to tumble and exit out of line with the point of entry.

DEBRIS AND EXIT WOUNDS

A bullet entering the body will usually carry particles of clothing and anything else that it penetrated before entering the body. In addition, the bullet may dislodge and carry bone fragments and muscle tissue fragments as it continues through the wound track. These contaminants can enlarge the exit wound and will inevitably cause infection if not removed. If the bullet does not exit the body, the bullet and this debris will remain at the end of the wound track. Whenever treating a bullet wound victim, the first aider must always examine the opposite side for an exit wound. There have been cases where an entry wound was treated while the victim bled out through an unnoticed exit wound in the back.

IMPERATIVE

With the above in mind, it is important to gather as much information about the weapon and the ammunition as possible to aid the medical providers. Other than obvious graze-wounds, there is no such thing as a minor bullet wound. Any bullet wound must be considered life-threatening and requiring the fastest access to professional care.

Managing Gunshot Wounds

As with all soft-tissue injuries, the first priority is to control any severe bleeding with direct pressure, hemostatic dressings, and, if necessary, application of a tourniquet. If the bullet has penetrated the thorax and created a sucking chest wound, the hole must be sealed to prevent the development of a pneumothorax. Packing the wound with sterile gauze or better yet, hemostatic gauze, can be effective in control of bleeding. Be sure to check for an exit wound and seal both openings. If the wound is to an extremity (arm or leg), apply a splint to prevent further damage. Treat the patient for shock before signs appear. Transport the patient to professional medical care as soon as possible.

Hemostatic plunger devices that inject hemostatic pellets directly into the wound to stop external and internal bleeding have been proven to outperform combat gauze. The Celox™-A applicator sells for under twenty-five dollars and should be included in the medical kit of anyone anticipating gunshot-related incidents.

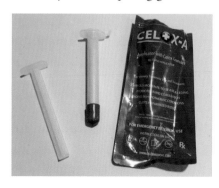

This hemostatic granule injector is specifically designed to seal bullet wounds and has saved lives. The injector is inserted to the depth of the wound and then slowly extracted while injecting the hemostatic material for the length of the wound.

Bullet Extraction

Bullet removal is far beyond first aid and any Good Samaritan protection and should only be attempted in the gravest extreme situations, when no access to professional medical care can be anticipated. No attempt to remove a bullet should be made for bullets that have entered the skull, thoracic cavity, or abdominal cavity. Bullets may be extracted if the bullet wound is shallow and the bullet is visible, the bullet has only penetrated the fatty or muscle tissue, or the bullet is in an extremity. A bullet may have penetrated or nicked an artery and be the only thing preventing severe bleeding. Consider this possibility if the wound is in the thigh, shoulder, or upper arm.

PREPARATION FOR BULLET EXTRACTION

1. Any bullet extraction will be extremely painful to the patient. If prescription pain relievers are available, administer them; if not, a combination of two Tylenol and three Aleve tablets have equivalent pain relief to codeine.
2. Have at least one assistant to hold the patient down.
3. Clean the area around the wound with surgical wipes or soap and water.
4. Have plenty of sterile bandages on hand.
5. Boil all instruments to sterilize them. If not practical, use a flame.
6. Wear sterile surgical gloves and a surgical mask or equivalent.
7. Have a syringe or bulb syringe with sterile water to flush the wound.
8. Be sure that the patient is not showing signs of shock, as attempting this procedure will only worsen the condition.

REMOVAL OF BULLET

1. If the bullet wound is shallow, palpate the skin to locate it.
2. If the bullet is not visible, flush the wound and use a flashlight to attempt to see it.
3. If it is too deep to visualize, slowly insert a sterile probe to determine how deep the bullet is located. Be sure you are contacting the bullet and not a bone or bone fragment.
4. Slowly insert a sterile pair of long tweezers, hemostat, or (if medical equipment is not available) needle-nose pliers.

5. Once the bullet is felt, open the device just enough to grip the bullet.
6. Firmly grip the bullet and slowly pull it from the wound.
7. If the bullet has deformed, mushroomed, or turned, it may catch on the skin at the wound site, requiring some manipulation or even a small cut to free it.
8. Thoroughly flush the wound with sterile water and bandage.
9. Use hemostatic dressings, hemostatic injectors, or tourniquets if severe bleeding results.
10. Treat the patient for shock.
11. Administer antibiotics if available.

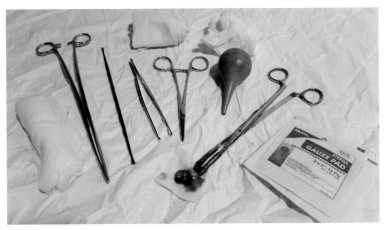

Bullet probe, various instruments, gauze, and a bulb-syringe to flush the wound. If antibiotics are available and the bullet has penetrated only muscle and fat tissue, bullets can be extracted, but when bullets have impacted organs and/or major blood vessels, prompt, professional, surgical intervention is critical.

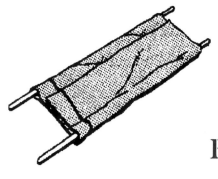

CHAPTER 27
EXPLOSION BLAST INJURIES

The increasing instability of society and the combination of foreign and domestic terrorist bombings creates the potential for the citizen first aider to be a victim or responder to an explosion and the resulting injuries. In addition, natural accidental explosions from natural gas and stored chemicals are a frequent, secondary effect of disasters and civil disorder.

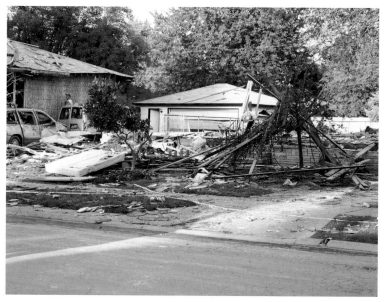

This house exploded as a result of flooding that floated the gas dryer away from the wall, breaking the gas line. The explosion occurred after the water had receded, when a security light timer caused a spark. Fortunately, no one was nearby. Note that adjoining houses were also severely damaged. Know how and where to shut off the gas and have a wrench nearby.

Scene Safety First

While scene safety and personal protection are always priorities when approaching an injury scene, they must be the primary concern after a bomb or explosion incident. After the initial blast, a number of hazards are created that further endanger the safety and health of the initial victims and the responding first aiders. These hazards must be considered and mitigated before effective triage and care can be provided.

In the case of a deliberate, man-made explosion, such as a terrorist bombing, it is not improbable that a second bomb may be detonated intentionally to harm and kill first responders, or the criminals may follow up the initial blast by initiating an active-shooter operation against survivors, responders, and bystanders. It may be advisable to carefully observe the scene from a safe distance, and/or await the arrival of police to provide security, before attempting to provide care. Some hazards to consider include the following:

+ The explosion may be part of a civil disorder or crime event, and the first aider may be assaulted or shot at by rioters or looters. Careful evaluation of the risks should precede entry into this type of environment regardless of good intentions. Being armed or having armed security may be justified to rescue and aid injured and endangered victims.

+ Explosions may rupture gas lines and puncture containers of flammable liquids, creating the potential for secondary explosions or flash fires. Rapid extrication of victims may take precedent over all other medical considerations in such cases.

+ Electrical lines may be broken or damaged, creating the potential for victim and responder electrocution. Be observant for downed power lines, exposed wires, or potentially charged water or metal objects.

+ An explosion and building collapse may free asbestos and other toxic materials into the air as dust and mist. Adequate respiratory protection is especially important in post-blast environments.

+ The violence of a large blast can leave unstable walls, sharp protrusions, and weakened floors and stairways. Further collapses can injure or trap the incautious first aider. Observe and analyze the victim's location and your entry and extrication route. Wait for help or try to shore-up hazards before entry.

Personal Protection

While latex gloves and a face mask may be sufficient personal protection for response to normal injuries and illnesses, they are inadequate for the extreme hazards generated by an explosion. The well-prepared first aider should have a hard hat; heavy, leather-palmed gloves; safety goggles; and a certified N95 dust/mist respirator. The World Trade Center attack in 2001 is a good example of the immediate and long-term consequences of inadequate scene safety and personal protection on responders.

Explosion-Generated Injuries

The unique quality of explosions is that they can generate a large number of patients with a large number of injuries instantly. The first responder/first aider can be faced with one or more patients with the following:

+ One or more sites of arterial bleeding
+ One or more serious lacerations
+ One or more amputations
+ One or more areas of first-, second-, and third-degree burns
+ One or more abdominal wounds or eviscerations
+ One or more sucking chest wounds
+ One or more single, multiple, closed, or open fractures
+ A collapsed lung due to pneumothorax or hemothorax
+ Airway obstruction
+ Cardiac arrest
+ Head and brain injuries
+ Hazardous chemical exposure
+ Shock

A thorough search should be conducted to be sure that all injured victims have been found. As always: treat life-threatening injuries (severe bleeding, sucking chest wounds) and life-threatening conditions (cardiac arrest, airway obstruction, respiratory arrest) first. Extricate only if the patient is in danger in the location they are found. Triage and treat based on seriousness of the injuries. Take special care to avoid movement and protect the cervical spine, as blasts are more likely to cause head, brain, and spinal injuries.

The Effects of Blast Overpressure

Overpressure is a unique source of injury from explosions. Large explosions such as what might result from a van or truck bomb can create a pressure wave sufficient to cause internal injuries. An explosion sufficient to collapse buildings can generate a 5 psi overpressure that will rupture eardrums. A bigger blast with a 15 psi overpressure can cause lung damage and even a closed pneumothorax, requiring a needle decompression procedure. Very large explosions such as those generated by loads of ammonium nitrate or nuclear devices can generate pressures in excess of 30 psi, where those not killed by flying debris or being thrown through the air will die from the overpressure.

Safe Standoff Distances for Bombs

The table below shows the US Department of Transportation recommended safe distances for various sizes of bombs.

Threat Description	Explosive Capacity	Minimum Standoff Distance	Preferred Standoff Distance	Shelter in Place Zone
Pipe Bomb	5 lbs.	70 ft.	1,200 ft.	71–1,950 ft.
Suicide Vest	20 lbs.	110 ft.	1,700 ft.	111–1,699 ft.
Briefcase Bomb	50 lbs.	150 ft.	1,850 ft.	151–1,849 ft.
Car Bomb	500 lbs.	325 ft.	1,900 ft.	391–1,899 ft.
Van Bomb	1,000 lbs.	400 ft.	2,400 ft.	401–2,399 ft.
Box Truck Bomb	4,000 lbs.	640 ft.	3,800 ft.	641–3,799 ft.
Semi-Trailer Bomb	10–60,000 lbs.	1,575 ft.	9,500 ft.	1,571–9,299 ft.

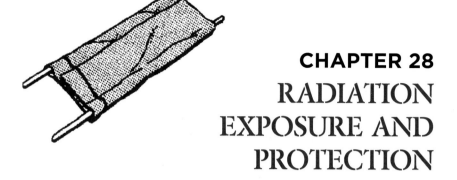

CHAPTER 28
RADIATION EXPOSURE AND PROTECTION

W hile massive nuclear war remains a possibility, more limited nuclear events and conflicts have become far more probable. The most probable sources of public exposure to radiation today are listed below.

+ Single or multiple nuclear power plant meltdowns such as those seen at Fukushima and Chernobyl. Such events could result in regional contamination in major population areas.

+ Terrorist initiation of a limited nuclear detonation, dirty-bomb, or covert spreading of radioactive material in public places. Such events would limit exposure to a limited number of people in a limited area.

+ Limited nuclear wars overseas. India vs. Pakistan, Israel vs. Iran, China vs. Russia all are potential scenarios where a few or even dozens of nuclear weapons could be detonated. Fallout would travel westward to the United States. Limiting any exposure, particularly in the first weeks and months after such an event, would definitely be prudent.

The above scenarios could result in significant incidents of radiation sickness, as well as increased cancer risk. These scenarios would also create significant survival challenges due to civil disorder, grid failure, and overwhelmed health and safety agencies, leaving the citizens to initiate their own protective and medical aid initiatives.

Radioactivity Exposure and Its Effects
The table below provides the estimated effects of radiation exposure. Note that even without the benefit of knowing the dosage, how soon the symptoms appear and how many people in the same area are affected is a good indication of developing disability and fatality rates.

Be aware that disability and death rates may vary widely depending on the health and age of the exposed persons. The lower exposures (50–120 roentgens) might be anticipated from distant events such as overseas nuclear exchanges or nuclear power plant accidents. Being close to or downwind of a nuclear detonation or power plant melt-down could result in exposures from 100 to 300 roentgens, depending on distance and how long you spent in the contaminated area. Higher exposures would be limited to those directly in or near a nuclear detonation or detonations. Of course, any exposure can increase your potential for cancer, leukemia, and a host of other medical issues in the future. It is particularly important to protect children and adolescents from any level of exposure because it is more likely to cause illness and birth defects years and decades later.

Expected Effects of Short-Term Gamma Radiation Exposure

Acute Dose (Roentgens)	Anticipated Effects of Radiation Exposure
0–50	No obvious symptoms. Possible minor blood changes.
60–120	Vomiting, nausea will affect about 5 to 10 percent of exposed personnel within 24 hours of exposure. Some fatigue may occur, but no disability or deaths anticipated.
130–170	Vomiting, nausea will affect about 25 percent of exposed personnel within about one day. This may be followed with other symptoms of radiation sickness, but no deaths can be anticipated.
180–220	Vomiting, nausea will affect about 50 percent of exposed personnel within about one day. This will be followed with other symptoms of radiation sickness, but no deaths can be anticipated.
270–330	Vomiting, nausea will affect nearly all exposed personnel on the first day. This will be followed with other symptoms of radiation sickness. Prolonged recovery time and 20 percent deaths within 2–6 weeks can be anticipated.
400–500	Vomiting and nausea will affect all exposed personnel within the first day of exposure. Severe symptoms of radiation sickness will last months and 50 percent of exposed personnel will die.
550–750	Vomiting and nausea will affect all exposed personnel within 4 hours of exposure. Severe symptoms of radiation sickness. Few survivors and prolonged convalescence time for those who survive.
1,000 >	Vomiting and nausea will affect all exposed personnel within a few hours of exposure. Few or no survivors from radiation sickness.
5,000 >	All exposed personnel incapacitated almost immediately. 100 percent fatalities within one week.

RULE OF THUMB FOR ESTIMATION OF TOTAL DOSAGE ACCUMULATED

D = Dosage in roentgens
I = Intensity of roentgens per hour
T = Time of exposure in hours
D = I x T

For example: If the dosage rate is found to be 70 roentgens per hour and you have been exposed for 3 hours, it is 70 x 3 = 210 roentgens accumulated dosage.

Nuclear detonations or accidents will result in the production of radioactive fallout. Fallout is simply radioactive particulates and fine dust thrown upwards by the blast. Since the heavier particles fall first, they start falling downwind closest and soonest after the blast. This makes these particles the most dangerous. The finer dust will fall further downwind over days and weeks following the initial blast. All radioactive fallout is subject to decay in radiation, so it is most dangerous within the first hours and days after it is created but continues to radiate at a declining rate for years and decades.

In the event of a so-called dirty bomb or the covert spreading of radioactive materials by terrorists, the radiation levels may vary widely, and the exposure areas will be limited to a few buildings or a few blocks. Those who may have aspirated radioactive particulates or unknowingly spent extended time in contaminated areas may develop varying levels of radiation sickness.

What Is Radiation?

Fallout particles can range from sand-like particles falling close to the source of a nuclear event to very fine dust that travels hundreds of miles from the source. There are three sources of radiation exposure from fallout.

+ Alpha particles cannot penetrate unbroken skin, but if ingested from contaminated food or drinks or inhaled from fallout in the air, they can reach unprotected internal organs and have serious effects.

+ Beta particles can cause beta-burns if left on unprotected skin and can cause more serious damage if ingested or inhaled.

✚   Both alpha and beta exposure hazards can be reduced by washing or dusting off particulates and wearing an effective mask.

✚   Gamma rays are like x-rays in that they can penetrate most materials with ease. These rays pass through the body, damaging cells and vital organs. The more intense the gamma radiation is and the longer the time of exposure, the more severe the damage. In addition to keeping particulates out of and off of your body, you must act to get out of the contaminated area as quickly as possible and thoroughly decontaminate yourself once out of the area. All clothing and equipment exposed to fallout must be abandoned or decontaminated.

Fallout shelters use massive amounts of soil, concrete, and other materials to reduce the amount of gamma radiation that penetrates the shelter. Additional filtering of air reduces the amount of gamma radiating material that enters the shelter. The more time you spend in such a shelter or even within a massive building or basement, the less your exposure will be. However, if the area of contamination is limited, such as downwind of a nuclear power plant, prompt evacuation and decontamination, if practical, would be far more effective than remaining in the contaminated area in any kind of shelter.

Signs and Symptoms of Radiation Sickness

Radiation sickness results from the damage that gamma rays do to the cells and organs of the body. How soon the signs and symptoms appear and how severe they are is a good indication of exposure rates and potential mortality. Initial symptoms include nausea, irritability, vomiting, diarrhea, and general fatigue. These symptoms may disappear after a few days but reappear within one to two weeks along with more serious symptoms of hair loss, hemorrhaging, and bleeding under the skin. Compromised immune systems will result in fever, infections, and disability. Vomiting, diarrhea, and internal hemorrhaging results in severe dehydration. The sooner these symptoms appear after exposure, the lower the survival rate will be. Radiation sickness is not contagious. Decontaminated victims cannot "infect" family members or caregivers.

If you are exposed to radioactive fallout, do the following:

+ Get out of the contaminated area as fast as you can to reduce total exposure rates.
+ Put on a dust mask or improvise a respirator from dampened cloth immediately to keep particles out of the body.
+ Dust off any contamination on your clothing.
+ If possible, don rain ponchos, rain suits, plastic bags, or other waterproof and dust proof clothing. Be sure to have your head covered to keep particles out of your hair.
+ Once out of the contaminated area, carefully remove contaminated outer garments. Dust and wash (spray or shower) skin, hair, feet/shoes, etc. as thoroughly as possible. Remove the mask last. Leave contaminated clothing and material well away from shelter.
+ Decontaminate any food cans, utensils, and equipment before use.
+ If available, take potassium iodide pills or liquid per dosage instructions. Note: Overdosing on potassium iodide can be harmful, so follow instructions.

Treating Radiation Poisoning

In addition to preventive use of potassium iodine tablets there are other measures you can take to improve your survival chances and shorten recovery time.

+ Maintain hydration with vitamin- and electrolyte-fortified water. When and if oral hydration cannot be tolerated, the use of intravenous fluids or fluid enemas may be necessary.
+ Strong iron supplements should be given to combat severe anemia and weakness.
+ Antibiotics should be given at the first signs of fever or infection as the immune system may not be able to fend off even minor illness or wound infections.
+ Burns and wounds must be treated with special care to avoid any kind of contamination.
+ Since internal bleeding often occurs in radiation poisoning, aspirin should be avoided.
+ Milk of Magnesia or Pepto-Bismol may be used to reduce diarrhea and vomiting.

Radioactive Decay and the Rule of Sevens

Although heavily radiated areas such as near Chernobyl can be unsafe for decades or even centuries, most contaminated areas will become safer as time passes. This is because of radioactive decay. Simply put: radioactivity declines by a factor of ten for every sevenfold increase in time after the initial event. This is known as the "rule of sevens." So after seven hours, the residual fission radioactivity declines 90 percent, to one-tenth its level at 1 hour. After 7x7 hours (49 hours, approx. 2 days), the level drops again by 90 percent. So now it's just 1 percent of the lethal dosage it was after one hour. After 7x2 days (two weeks) it drops a further 90 percent, and so on. After 14 weeks the rate drops even faster.

Respiratory Protection

Ninety percent of the immediate harm from radioactive fallout is from inhalation and ingestion of the contaminant. Skin and hair exposure must be decontaminated as soon as possible, but what you have breathed and swallowed will do irreversible harm. Fortunately, the N95 dust/mist respirator sold in most hardware stores for painting is all the protection you need from nuclear fallout. These masks cost less than $2 each. They also can protect you from chemical-contaminated dust and soot created by bombs, fires, and storms. These masks are small and light enough to carry everywhere. You should have at least one in every jacket, purse, glove box, briefcase, and pack, and have more of them at home. The mask will keep contaminated air and mists out of your lungs and will keep radioactive dust particles out of your body, where alpha and beta radiation do the most harm. So your most important and effective step to protection is stocking up on N95 masks. Aim to have at least one with you and every family member wherever you go.

It is critical that you keep masks in a sealed plastic bag so that it is not pre-contaminated before you put it on. It is also critical that you fit it properly according to the instructions on the package. Air and contaminants will not go through a filter if they can go around them. Be aware that all bets are off if you have a beard or heavy facial hair. You may want to consider packing a plastic razor with the mask.

Protective Clothing

Having kept the hazardous material out of the body, we can move on to how to keep it *off* of the skin and hair. There are three situations where body protection may be necessary:

1. Situations where heavy biological contamination exists, such as hospitals, in the presence of dead bodies, or in areas where biological agents have been dispersed.
2. Situations where airborne chemical contaminants are present, such as downwind of a chemical spill or in building debris.
3. Any area in the downwind "footprint" of fallout from a nuclear detonation for at least two weeks.

Fortunately, there are fairly simple and easy solutions available. You do not need heavy NBC (nuclear, biological, chemical) suits and masks. These products are designed for the military and industry to fight and work for extended periods in high-risk environments. You just need immediate protection long enough to get out of the contaminated area or reach a fallout shelter.

You can improvise a protective suit from plastic bags, rubber bands, and a pair of surgical gloves. Latex gloves are a handy item to keep with each mask. Such an improvised suit would consist of two large bags used as a skirts and head/body cover and four small ones used to cover arms, legs and shoes. It is important to note that any form of non-porous covering is better than none. Even just the one big bag covers fifty percent of the body. A raincoat or poncho is far better than nothing.

A step better is the basic Tyvek™ chemical protective suits with hoods and feet. These are cheap (around $12), light, and easy to carry. These too are often available in hardware stores and are used by painters. They are a bit bulky for pockets but fit well in a glove box, desk drawer, or locker.

Internal Organ Protection

Potassium iodide is a specific blocker of thyroid radioiodine uptake. Taking potassium iodide effectively prevents the thyroid gland from being saturated with harmful radioiodine from fallout contamination that can lead to cancer. Fourteen 130-mg potassium iodide pills sell for about $20. The government has stockpiles of these pills for distribution, but having your own supply is highly advisable.

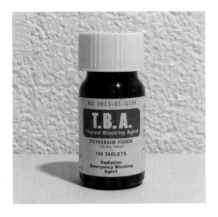

Potassium iodide tablets can be taken to block absorption of radioactive iodine to vital organs.

Decontamination

Now that we have kept the bad stuff off our skin and out of our lungs, we need to be able to remove contamination and contaminated coverings without transferring it back into and onto our bodies. This process is called decontamination. Of course, we want to do this when we are outside of the danger zone or at the entrance to more effective shelter (underground for fallout, enclosed from biological or chemical) locations. Ideally this is a two-person job, with both wearing protective clothing. It should be done in a location that will not permit contaminated run-off, spray mists, or dusts to contaminate other safe areas.

There are five steps to effective decontamination:

1. Gross decontamination involves simply brushing off or rinsing off any surface contaminants as well as dumping any contaminated gear that will not be needed.

2. Thorough decontamination is accomplished using pressurized water (not high pressure) with a neutralizing or disinfecting solution. Soap and water will clear most chemical and fallout materials. Plain water used copiously will be less effective but may be adequate. The best device for spraying is a commercial pump garden sprayer. Keep a clean one handy at home. They are also good for fighting small class "A" fires and general hygiene tasks.

3. Next you need to "peel off" the protective clothing, minimizing any contact with the clean clothing and skin underneath. Step out of the foot coverings onto an uncontaminated surface. Remove the face mask and then peel off the gloves

following standard personal protection degloving procedure. At no time should the hand contact the outside of the glove.

4. If any clothing was potentially contaminated before you put on the protection, it must be removed, and any skin or hair must be rewashed before dressing and entering the safe zone or shelter.

5. Finish by bagging all contaminated materials and containing all contaminated waters. Be sure to decontaminate well away from areas that you may need to use, as these locations are now contaminated until radioactive decay reduces the radiation levels.

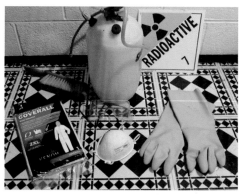

Basic, hooded, chemical (painters) coveralls, rubber gloves, dust respirators, and goggles are all that is needed to keep fallout dust off. A brush can get most of the dust off prior to removal, but hosing down with soap and water is best. A simple garden sprayer is excellent for decontamination of chemical, biological, and radioactive contaminants.

Radiation Burns

Sunburns are, in fact, radiation burns. Radiation burns can also result from exposure to the flash of radiation emitted from a nuclear explosion. While the burns themselves can be treated like any other first- or second-degree burns, the exposure to this direct radiation will also cause radiation poisoning. The level of poisoning will depend on the closeness of the blast source and the amount of tissue exposed. Beta burns are caused by beta particles (fallout) on the skin surface. The beta radiation causes shallow surface burns only. Beta radiation can be stopped by most clothing. Inhaled or ingested beta particles can cause internal burns and beta burns to the eyes can be particularly damaging. Therefore, an N95 mask and goggles along with full-body covering is always recommended for fallout protection. Frequent brushing off or washing off dust will prevent beta burns.

Radiation Detection Instruments

If radiation is a serious concern, a radiation detection instrument may be a worthwhile investment. There are a lot of reasonably priced older dosimeters and survey meters on sale at preparedness shows and on the internet. Uncalibrated radiation detectors sell for about $20 because the calibration radiation sources used for this procedure are so strictly regulated, but there are sources to have them calibrated. Calibrated survey meters sell for about $80 and new ones sell for about $150. Go to www.sportsmansguide.com or www.colmans.com for these items. There are also more modern nuclear radiation detectors and monitors on the market. These range in price from $180 to over $300. Regardless of calibration, any detected exposure level ranges or area radiation above normal is cause for concern and precautions.

Dosimeters are intended to be worn in the pocket and checked frequently to determine how much radiation the wearer has been exposed to. They come with a charger and instructions. A charger and two dosimeters sell for about $40.

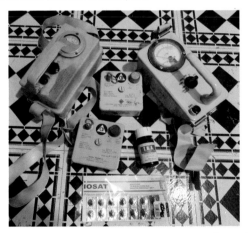

Surplus civil defense survey meters can be purchased at preparedness shows and on the internet at reasonable costs. Some are calibrated and others are not, but calibration services are also available. CD V-742 pocket dosimeters and CD V-750 chargers are also still available. These are used to register personal exposure rather than area radiation.

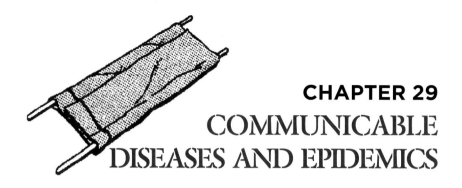

CHAPTER 29
COMMUNICABLE DISEASES AND EPIDEMICS

Communicable Diseases

While not all communicable diseases become epidemics or pandemics, they all pose a hazard to those rendering first aid to the ill and injured. Disaster conditions inherently create greater risk of the development and spread of communicable disease. Many of the worst epidemics and pandemics have developed in the wake of war, revolution, and large-scale disaster. Prior to the development of vaccinations and effective sanitation practices, more soldiers died of diseases than from combat. There are four ways that diseases can be transmitted to humans:

+ Contact transmission. Direct contact transmission is from one infected person to another uninfected person through actual touching. Indirect contact transmission occurs when an infected person contaminates an inanimate object and then another person touches that object and acquires the pathogen.

+ Airborne transmission. As the name implies, airborne transmission is carried in the air, typically from an infected person's coughs or sneezes. Infected droplets carry the pathogen to be inhaled by others.

+ Vehicle transmission. In this case, the pathogen is introduced into the body through contaminated food, water, fluids, or blood.

+ Vector transmission. Typical vector transmissions are from mosquito bites (e.g., malaria), ticks (e.g., Rocky Mountain spotted fever), and animal bites (e.g., rabies).

The chances of developing an infection from exposure to a communicable disease is dependent on three factors.

1. The amount (dose) present in the environment and source of the pathogen.

2. The extent to which the pathogen survives on surfaces when exposed to air and light. This is known as virulence. The virulence of pathogens differs greatly, from a few hours to many days.

3. The individual's resistance to infection. People with weakened immune systems, poor nutrition, or preexisting medical conditions may become ill while healthier individuals may not.

The best protection against airborne transmitted pathogens is the proper wearing of an N95 respirator whenever there is the potential for exposure. The best protection against contact transmission is the wearing and proper removal of latex gloves. It is best to wear gloves, an N95 respirator, and eye or face protection to guard against contact, airborne, and vector-borne pathogens when rendering aid to any patient. Particular cautions should be followed when exposed to those with a fever, diarrhea, draining wounds, or jaundiced (yellow) skin as these are definitive signs of many communicable diseases. Thorough handwashing; the careful disposal of contaminated gloves, respirators, and equipment; and decontamination of exposed surfaces is critical to avoiding infection.

Common Communicable Diseases

Hepatitis is caused by chemicals, alcohol, drugs, and viruses. Hepatitis A is more commonly seen in children and does not have any serious complications. Hepatitis B is caused by a virus and is transmitted through blood, saliva, or sexual contact. This virus is extremely hardy and can remain virulent on surfaces for six weeks or more. The symptoms of Hepatitis B include nausea, vomiting, fatigue, and abdominal pain. Non-A/Non-B hepatitis is usually associated with blood transfusions.

Herpes is a common and usually mild infection caused by the herpes simplex virus (HSV). It can cause cold sores on the mouth or face (oral herpes) as well as symptoms around the genitals and thighs (genital herpes). Herpetic whitlow is a related and incurable viral infection that can be contracted when the first aider has a break in the skin and the breach comes into contact with sores or oral secretions from an infected patient. A first aider with any kind of cut or scratch on the hands should double glove.

Meningitis is an inflammation of the brain covering (meninges) that is usually transmitted through contaminated food or water. This disease is serious and often deadly, killing about 500 people per year in the United States. The symptoms include sudden high fever, sudden headache, stiff neck, vomiting, nausea, sleepiness, confusion, shivering, light sensitivity, convulsions, and a deep purple rash. In addition to full personal protective equipment, thorough decontamination procedures must be initiated. All potentially contaminated food and water sources must be avoided.

Tuberculosis is contagious but not communicable unless the patient is coughing or creating infected droplets. There must be direct contact with the patient's sputum to be infected. However, since this disease is serious, respiratory and eye protection is advisable for first aiders if tuberculosis is suspected.

Acquired Immune Deficiency Syndrome (AIDS) is caused by a virus (human immunodeficiency virus, or HIV) that attacks cells in the immune system. The loss of these cells renders the victim highly susceptible to many diseases. Symptoms of AIDS include severe fatigue, night sweats, skin lesions, weight loss, swollen lymph nodes, and even dementia. The AIDS infection can be transmitted through blood, semen, and vaginal secretions, but not through general contact or oral contact. Blood-borne pathogen (BBP) protection, including gloves, eye protection, respiratory protection, and hand washing, should be implemented whenever contact with blood is involved in rendering first aid.

Epidemics and Pandemics

Epidemics and pandemics may become more frequent and severe due to increased population densities and international travel. They can also be the secondary result of civil unrest, the breakdown of sanitation services, shortages, and economic chaos. Even a cyber-attack, electromagnetic pulse, or grid failure could lead to a pandemic and, of course, there is the potential for a deliberate distribution of pathogens by terrorists or hostile nations. New pathogens are emerging every year, and it is inevitable that some will prove to be highly contagious and deadly. With that in mind, let's review viral diseases in general and some of the methods for prevention and treatment of viral diseases.

Viruses are much smaller than bacteria and are made up of a material with an exterior protein. Viruses cannot make their own protein like most other cells, and therefore are dependent on a host for survival.

Each virus targets a specific body organ such as the lungs, liver, or even the blood. Viruses are not affected by antibiotics. The best protection against viruses is a strong immune system and good personal hygiene. While some viruses—such as measles, rubella, mumps, smallpox, and polio—are preventable through vaccination, others are not. Vaccinations for various forms of flu and pneumonia are only partially effective. The following is only a partial list of the most common viruses:

+ Influenza
+ Chickenpox
+ HIV
+ Ebola
+ Polio
+ Mumps
+ Hepatitis
+ Shingles
+ Lyme disease
+ Smallpox
+ Measles
+ Herpes
+ Some types of colds
+ Coronaviruses

Viruses can be transmitted from contact with infected animals such as birds, pigs, bats, rodents, dogs, and horses. Other viruses can be transmitted from animal bites, and insect bites such as those of ticks, flies, fleas, mosquitos, and lice. Human transmission can result from skin contact, oral contact, sexual contact, and close respiratory contact, such as coughing. Viruses can survive in air for as long as three hours and on surfaces for two to three days.

Vitamins for Prevention and Treatment

It has been found that low levels of Vitamin D3 resulted in increased vulnerability to cold and flu. A strong correlation has been found between those with TB, and hepatitis C, and Vitamin D3 deficiencies. Vitamin D3 helps the body make an antibiotic protein called cathelicidin that is known to kill viruses, fungi, parasites, and bacteria. During flu season (or during an epidemic) it is recommended to take 50,000 IU daily for five days and then 5,000 to 10,000 IU daily thereafter.

More than thirty clinical studies have confirmed the antiviral effects of Vitamin C against a wide range of flu viruses. Vitamin C inactivates the virus while strengthening the immune system's ability to resist the virus. The general recommendation is an oral dose of 10,000 mg daily, but some stronger viruses (like coronavirus) may require intravenous doses as high as 100,000 to 150,000 mg. If IV vitamin C is not available, a gradual increase of oral Vitamin C up to 50,000 mg may be possible before bowel tolerance is reached.

Herbal Remedies

A variety of studies have shown that some herbal remedies are effective against some viruses. Elderberry can be effective against influenza A and B. Astragulus root is effective against the Coxsackie B virus. Licorice root has been used to treat hepatitis C and HIV. Olive leaf has been proven effective in the treatment of flu, colds, hepatitis C, malaria, gonorrhea, and tuberculosis.

Other foods that may be effective in prevention and treatment of viral infections include:

+ Wild blueberries
+ Sprouts
+ Cilantro
+ Coconut oil
+ Garlic
+ Ginger
+ Sweet potatoes
+ Turmeric
+ Kale
+ Parsley
+ Red clover
+ Elderberry

Non-Viral Infections

It is important to keep in mind that while most epidemic pathogens are viral and not affected by antibiotics, other non-viral pathogens such as streptococcus, salmonella, E. coli, tuberculosis, cholera, and bubonic plague may beset the infected victim, who may have a weakened immune system, be undernourished, or have been exposed to poor sanitation. For this reason, antibiotics should still be kept available. Antibiotics are available from pet supply stores, fish supply stores, and survival supply outlets. These are exactly the same products as are prescribed for humans, but at a much lower price without any prescription required. It is advisable to maintain a supply of these, but they are not to be used for viral infections.

Self-prescribed and obtained antibiotics should be used only when no other alternative is available and serious infections and diseases are evident or imminent. Antibiotics are most effective against various types of plague pathogens that could be the primary source of an epidemic and against many secondary infections common in disasters. Dosage information can be obtained from the internet or the Merck Manual and based on the type of disease and patient. Yes, in some cases the survivor may be forced to guess and err on the side of more. Adult dosages of most antibiotics range from 250 mg to 500 mg every 6 to 10 hours. Dosage decreases with child ages.

Penicillin is the first antibiotic that was developed in 1928. It is also the longest and most over-used and some bacteria have become resistant to it. Penicillin is generally effective against common staphylococcus and streptococcus infections as well as clostridium and listeria genera. These common bacterial infections would be anticipated in open wounds and contaminated water and food during a long-running disaster. About 10 percent of the population may be allergic to penicillin.

Amoxicillin is effective in treating ear infections, strep throat, pneumonia, skin infections, urinary tract infections, and other types of bacterial infections. It also is used for some kinds of stomach

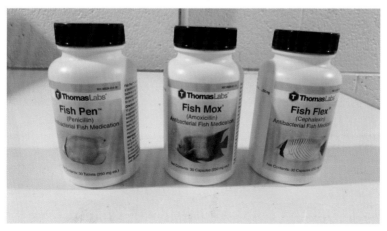

Bottles of antibiotics can be purchased from veterinary, aquarium, or survival-supply vendors.

infections. It has been used effectively for people exposed to anthrax. Its effectiveness against pneumonia and skin infections makes it an essential survival medication, since these infections are most common in disasters and nuclear events. Amoxicillin should not be given to those who are allergic to penicillin.

Cephalexin is effective against infections of the middle ear, bones, joints, skin, and urinary tract. It can also be used against certain kinds of pneumonia and strep throat. Cephalexin is not effective against methicillin-resistant staphylococcus known as MRSA.

Epidemics and Pandemics

An international pandemic is the most feared and most probable cataclysm facing civilization. Not even a nuclear war has the potential to obliterate civilization and exterminate most or all of the human race as does a highly communicable, incurable, and biologically devastating virus or bacteria. Such an event would be as devastating to civilized societies and the world economy as a nuclear war. The recent COVID-19 pandemic was not the one experts refer to as "the big one," and the fact that we have recently experienced a pandemic in no way reduces the probability of another, more devastating pandemic occurring in the next few years or decades. Overpopulation, urban concentration, and world travel have established the potential for rapid spread of pathogens faster than it would be possible to detect or isolate them. Paradoxically, improved sanitation and overuse of antibiotics has resulted in weakened immune systems in all of the more advanced countries. Massive immigration (legal and illegal) from so-called third-world and conflict-ridden countries brings previously rare disease closer to the world's great cities and civilizations. Laboratory experimentation, biological mutation, and even deliberate development can unleash new and more deadly strains of plagues upon a vulnerable population.

The most dangerous combination of properties for a pathogen would be a highly communicable pathogen with a long incubation period that could spread undetected for weeks before symptoms alerted the world to its presence. One with a long recovery time and/or a high mortality rate would certainly destroy civilization as we know it. In addition, the accidental, incidental, or deliberate initiation of a pandemic could be a secondary effect of a primary disaster. A financial collapse would cause strikes and civil disorder that could result in the interruption of sanitation systems, medical services, water purification, and food production and delivery. All of these open the door to communicable diseases. A nuclear war would result in radiation sickness that compromises the immune system and exhibits many of the symptoms of communicable diseases to begin with. A large-scale natural disaster, an electro-magnetic pulse (EMP), or a cyberattack on the power grid could also trigger a domino-effect that would lead to an epidemic.

COVID-19 Protection

While the mass vaccinations may have ended the initial COVID-19 pandemic, there is no reason to be complacent. So-called herd-immunity reduces the *probability* of exposure, not the *possibility* of exposure. A significant portion of the population may have chosen not to be vaccinated, it has not been established how long the efficacy of vaccinations will last, and other mutations of coronaviruses may emerge. Continued adherence to personal protection and sanitation protocols must be sustained at the first indications of an emerging contagion.

A regimen of high dose (8,000 units per day) zinc supplements and baby aspirin were found to reduce the risk of contracting COVID-19, hospitalization, the chances of being put on a ventilator, and recovery time. These supplements may be of value in management of future outbreaks caused by similar viruses.

Effects of Infectious Diseases and Biological Agents

I was unable to find any tables or charts that included all of the essential information about the most likely epidemic sources, so I created the tables below for your reference. Note that while radiation sickness is not a communicable disease, it is included for comparison of effects.

Disease / Agent	Typhus	Typhoid Fever	Encephalitis	Brucellosis
Infective	High	Moderate	High	High
Transmittable	None	Moderate	None	None
Incubation Period	6–15 days	7–12 days	5–15 days	7–60 days
Duration of Illness	14–60 days	14–60 days	7–60 days	14–60 days
Mortality Rate*	10–40%	10%	10–80%	2–10%
Vaccine Available	Yes	Yes	No	No
Antibiotics Effective**	Yes	?	No	?

(Continued on next page)

Disease / Agent	Typhus	Typhoid Fever	Encephalitis	Brucellosis
Typical Symptoms	Headache Chills High fever Muscle pain Swollen lymph nodes Skin rash Stupor	Headache Weakness Sweating Muscle pain Dry cough Abdominal pain Diarrhea or constipation Rash Swollen abdomen Delirium	Headache Fever Muscle and joint aches Fatigue Confusion and delirium Paralysis Double vision Hearing and speech difficulty Unconsciousness	Headache Fever Chills Sweating Weakness Muscle and back pain

Disease / Agent	Pneumonic Plague	Septicemic Plague	Bubonic Plague	Cholera
Infective	High	High	High	High
Transmittable	High	High	High	High
Incubation Period	2–5 days	2–5 days	2–5 days	2–5 days
Duration of Illness	7–30 days	7–30 days	7–30 days	10–60 days
Mortality Rate*	100%	100%	100%	5–75%
Vaccine Available	?	?	?	No
Antibiotics Effective**	Yes	Yes	Yes	?
Typical Symptoms	Fever Headache Weakness Chest pain Difficulty breathing Cough Pneumonia Bloody mucous	Fever Chills Abdominal pain Weakness Bleeding into skin and other organs Skin turns blue or black at toes, fingers, other parts of body	Fever Headache Weakness Painful and swollen lymph nodes	Diarrhea Dehydration Blue, dry skin Stomach cramps Muscle cramps Vomiting Weakness Low blood pressure

Disease / Agent	Smallpox	Anthrax	Yellow Fever	Hemorrhagic Fever
Infective	High	Moderate	Low	Yes
Transmittable	High	None	High	High
Incubation Period	7–16 days	1–5 days	1–5 days	2–3 days
Duration of Illness	12–24 days	3–5 days	7–30 days	20–60 days
Mortality Rate*	5–60%	100%	5- 40%	90%
Vaccine Available	Yes	Yes	Yes	No
Antibiotics Effective**	No	Yes	?	?

(Continued on next page)

Typical Symptoms	Fever Headaches Severe fatigue Severe back pain Vomiting Red lesions starting on face and hands and spreading to trunk Lesions turn to pitted weeping blister	Raised itchy bumps Swollen sore lymph nodes Nausea and vomiting Fever Headaches Bloody diarrhea Abdominal pain	ACUTE PHASE Fever Nausea Light sensitivity Dizziness Red eyes, face, tongue Chest pain Shortness of breath Fever Shock TOXIC PHASE Yellow skin Vomiting blood Bleeding from nose and mouth Brain dysfunction Liver and kidney damage	Headaches Capillary bleeding Fever Skin swelling and bleeding Bloody diarrhea Purple skin spots Low blood pressure Vomiting with blood Muscle and joint pain Shock
Disease / Agent	**Influenza**	**Dysentery**	**Radiation Sickness (Mild)**	**Radiation Sickness (Severe)**
Infective	Yes	Moderate	No	No
Transmittable	High	High	No	No
Incubation Period	2–3 days	2–3 days	On Contact	On Contact
Duration of Illness	7–15 days	10–50 days	7–30 days	6–12 months
Mortality Rate*	5%	15%	0–20%	50–100%
Vaccine Available	Yes	No	No	No
Antibiotics Effective**	No	?	?	?
Typical Symptoms	High fever Runny nose Vomiting Sore throat Cough Muscle pain Headache Diarrhea Fatigue Dehydration	Fever Diarrhea Dehydration Stomach cramps Muscle aches Rectal pain Vomiting Shock Delirium	Symptoms appear in only 10–50% of those exposed within 24 hours Vomiting Nausea Fatigue	Symptoms appear in more than 50% of those exposed on the day of exposure Vomiting Nausea Fatigue Hair loss dehydration Diarrhea Shock

* Mortality rates are highly dependent on the age and general health of the victims and on prompt available care.

** The effectiveness of antibiotics depends on the victim's condition and on how soon they are administered. In some cases, the antibiotics may not directly affect the disease, but may treat secondary infections and thereby improve the recovery rate.

Surviving a Contagious Disease Epidemic

Although they are not always listed specifically, almost all communicable diseases can cause nausea, vomiting, loss of appetite, sweating, and diarrhea. These conditions lead directly to severe dehydration that in turn results in organ failure and death if not treated. Maintaining good oral hydration and electrolyte balance in the early stages of these diseases is critical. Once the patient can no longer tolerate oral fluids and/or is unconscious, oral fluids must be avoided and only IV and rectal (fluid enemas) are feasible. Maintaining hydration and the use of antibiotics where effective can greatly reduce mortality rates for most diseases.

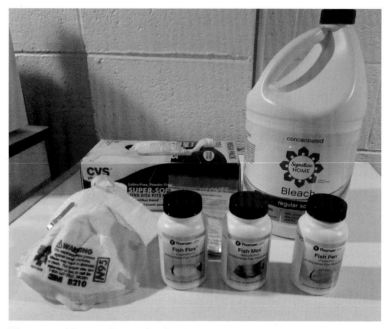

The use of latex gloves, hydration solutions, N95 respirators, bleach solutions, and available antibiotics could provide a significant advantage in surviving a large-scale epidemic

The single most effective defense against being infected is the ability to restrict or eliminate all contact with the population and sources of contamination as soon as possible. Once symptoms are detected and the word or rumor of an epidemic is spreading, you must be able to instantly isolate yourself and your family and remain isolated until the epidemic has burned itself out. Being able to hole-up in your home for four to eight weeks with enough food, water, medical supplies, fire extinguishers, defensive arms, and lighting and heating capacity is the only sure way to avoid becoming a victim of these deadly pathogens. The worst places to be are public transportation, grocery stores, hospitals, and disaster aid centers. If other potentially infected persons attempt to enter your home, you are justified in turning them away and using force if necessary to protect your own life and your family.

In a "worst case" situation where you are forced to evacuate your home or are unable to get to your home, you will need to have survival packs and skills that allow you to survive for an extended time without aid or contact with others. Water filtration, respiratory protection, safe food, and defensive arms will be especially important to survival in the open.

Anything and anyone coming into contact with you during an epidemic must be considered dangerous. Wearing N95 respirators when you are away from home or while caring for afflicted family members is essential. All water (regardless of sources) should be boiled for five minutes or treated with bleach at one quarter teaspoon per gallon. Wear latex gloves when handling any potentially contaminated items and use a spray of 10 percent bleach/water solution to decontaminate surfaces, canned goods, and any other potentially contaminated items from outside.

Most communities have plans for coping with a mass epidemic. There are stockpiles of antibiotics and medications ready for distribution, but civil disorder, infrastructure disruption, and other factors are sure to interfere with these efforts to some extent. Emergency volunteers and medical personnel will get these supplies first. How many of these people will be healthy, available, and ready to expose themselves and their families to a highly contagious and debilitating disease is difficult to estimate.

Summary

It can be anticipated that epidemics and pandemics will be part of the threat-matrix that modern, responsible citizens must prepare for. Government agencies and the health system will never be fully able to anticipate and react to new pathogens before they spread and affect the general population. High population densities combined with global travel and immigration guarantee even more lethal outbreaks in the future. Ultimately the individual citizen, family, and group must take strong independent preparatory and preventive action to survive the direct effects (illness) of an epidemic, but also the greater secondary effects on the economy and society. A few key preparedness and preventive actions are listed below.

✚ The ability to isolate yourself from human contact for 30 to 60 days is the most important and effective way to prevent exposure. This requires that you have sufficient water, food, fuel, medications, and other critical supplies in advance. This is sufficient for an immediate and passing emergency, but an extended and more lethal event could result in the need for far more well-developed and equipped survival and evacuation capacities.

✚ Maintaining general health, weight, and exercise habits greatly improves your chances of surviving any illness. Poor eating habits, lack of exercise, smoking, and neglected health maintenance is an invitation to infections.

✚ Always have plenty of N95 respirators, hand sanitizer, bleach, and disinfectants on hand.

✚ Good hygiene, including frequent hand washing, and avoidance of touching your face is important.

✚ Frequently clean all frequently touched surfaces such as doorknobs, railings, and tabletops with a household disinfectant.

✚ When away from home, clean hands before and after touching shopping carts, door handles, chair arms, money, and other frequently touched surfaces.

✚ Have a clean handkerchief to cover your mouth when you cough. Carrying a N95 folding respirator is advisable, as you could be caught in a closed space or in proximity to coughers.

✚ Avoid anyone who has flu-like symptoms or any location (e.g., schools, nursing homes, hospitals) where virus may be more prevalent.

✚ Avoid large gatherings and close proximity to groups, period.

✚ At the first sign of flu-like symptoms, seek medical help. Get tested and take aggressive treatment. The sooner treatment begins, the greater your survival chances will be.

✚ Support your immune system with supplemental doses of Vitamin C and Vitamin D3 as mentioned above.

CHAPTER 30
PATIENT PACKAGING AND TRANSPORT

U nder normal circumstances the movement of an injured or ill person should be left to the well-trained and equipped EMTs of an ambulance service. When emergency transportation is not available the first aider may need to employ expedient and improvised techniques to safely move a patient to a safe location or even all the way to a medical care facility. Employing these methods may be justified if the following conditions are met:

1. The patient is in a remote or wilderness location far from roads where an ambulance can be accessed.
2. The patient is in an area where continued hazards such as fire, hazardous fumes, cold, civil unrest, or other conditions necessitate long distance evacuation.
3. Nearby medical facilities and ambulance services are rendered unusable because of storm damage, violence, epidemics, or other factors.

Spinal Immobilization
Any violent trauma can result in damage to the cervical (neck) spine. Further movement of the head and neck can cause damage to the spinal cord and permanent paralysis. Extreme care must be taken to stabilize the head and neck prior to moving any patient. While finding a patient lying prone and face up and forward is ideal, a traumatic event such as a fall, vehicle accident, or assault, may leave the victim face down, on their side, or in any contorted and unnatural position. The victim will need to be moved to the neutral position to facilitate a thorough examination, assure an open airway, and align the cervical spine for stabilization prior to further movement. One first aider must apply gentle traction to the head while slowly

turning it to align with the body (face forward). If the body must be turned or moved, the gentle traction must be maintained and the head turned as the body is moved to maintain alignment. Once the body is aligned, prone or sitting, a cervical collar or improvised collar must be applied before releasing the head. In the absence of a cervical collar, towels or newspaper may be used to stabilize the cervical spine. (See Expedient Rescue chapter.)

Improvised Stretchers

If you seriously anticipate the need to move an injured person, you may want to invest in a military surplus stretcher such as the Swiss Army collapsible stretcher, but otherwise you may need to improvise. A door or a wide board can be used if nothing else is at hand. Blankets and shirts can also be modified to create adequate stretchers.

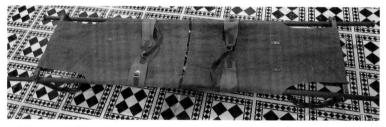

Military surplus stretchers are available at surplus outlets, but may be heavy and impractical for civilian use

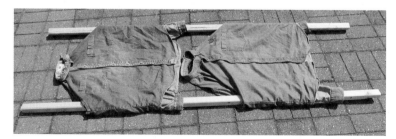

Two shirts can be used to create an improvised stretcher.

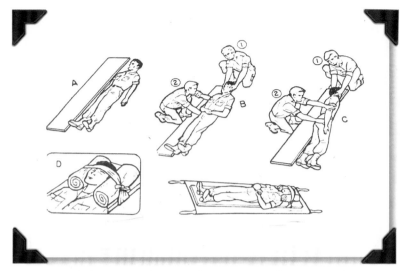

Even a wide board or door can be used as a litter. Note the person at the head maintaining spinal alignment, and how the head is secured in place prior to movement.

MAKING A BLANKET AND POLE STRETCHER

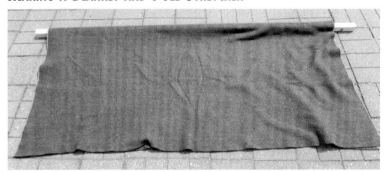

1 Blanket is doubled over a pole as shown.

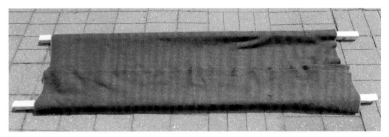

2 Fold the blanket halfway over the second pole as shown. The patient's weight will prevent the blanket from loosening.

Patient to Blanket Transfer

It is easier to transfer a prone patient onto a blanket than onto a stretcher, and a stretcher may not be available to those rendering emergency care under disaster conditions. Blankets are more commonly available, and once the patient is on a blanket, it is easy to lift the blanket and move them to a stretcher when available. A good quality wool blanket should be included in all first aid gear for use in treating shock, hypothermia, and for patient rescue and transport. The procedure for moving a patient to a blanket is as follows:

1. Position the blanket alongside the patient, making sure that the patient's head will be well supported when on the blanket. The lower legs may extend a bit over the end if necessary to provide room for the head.
2. C-fold about 6 inches of blanket on the side facing the patient. This will leave about 18 inches of blanket to roll and grip once the patient is centered.
3. Logroll the patient onto the side and pull the folded edges up against the patient.
4. Roll the patient back down into the prone position onto the blanket.
5. Pull the folded portion out. This should leave the patient approximately centered.
6. Each side of the blanket can now be rolled and gripped by one or more persons on each side.
7. Each lifter should be on one knee. On the count of 1-2-3, all lift together.
8. Note: If there is danger of cervical spine injury and enough people are available, a person at the patient's head should maintain spinal alignment throughout this procedure and be the one doing the counts and commands.

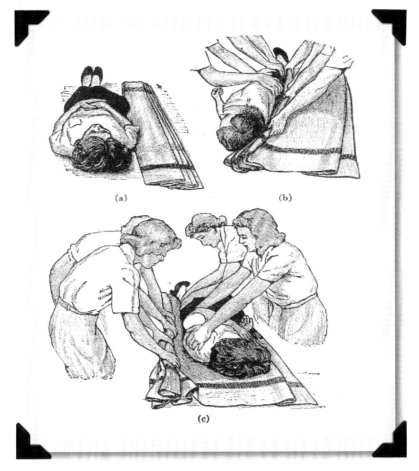

(a)　　　　　　　　(b)

(c)

Ideally, four people are needed to do a smooth transfer, but it can be done with just two. If the patient has suffered potential head and spinal injury, an additional person should hold traction on the head and maintain spinal alignment as the patient is turned.

Patient to Stretcher Transfer

Transferring an injured patient from the prone position to a stretcher must be done gently and while maintaining cervical spine alignment. Since it takes at least two people to carry a stretcher, the minimum number necessary to do the transfer is two. One person at the head holds the patient's head to preserve spinal alignment as the patient is rolled, and one person to logroll the victim onto their side to reach across and bring the stretcher close to the victim and then roll them back onto the stretcher. The person at the head is always in charge and does the count. One, two, three, the patient is rolled on their side. After the stretcher is in place: one, two, three, the patient rolled onto the stretcher.

Care must be taken to assure that the patient's head is far enough down to leave room for head stabilization and is close to the center-line of the stretcher to avoid the need to shift them after placement. Once the patient is on the stretcher they must be secured and padded for comfort and covered with a blanket. Even if a cervical collar is in place, the head must be stabilized with padding on both sides. The legs must be secured enough to assure that they do not shift and dangle in transport. The arms and hands should also be softly secured over the chest for safety. While two responders can manage this procedure, three or even four are better.

Carrying

Once the patient is secure, movement can be initiated. The route of carry should be scouted in advance and a plan for negotiating turns, obstacles, and stairs should be agreed upon. Lifting should be smooth and on a count of one, two, three. Once the carry has begun, the stretcher should remain level, and all tilting or bouncing must be avoided. If others are available, they may lead to clear the route or walk alongside for additional support. If a rest stop is necessary, select a safe, flat location, and gently lower the stretcher on the one, two, three count. The person at the head-end of the stretcher is responsible for constantly observing the patient and talking to them to assess his/her level of consciousness. Any group that anticipates moving patients should practice patient packaging and transport in advance.

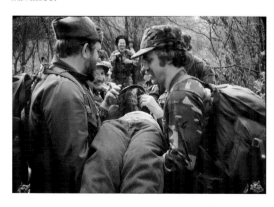

Survival trainees practice patient transport under realistic conditions.

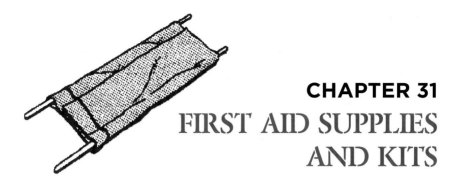

CHAPTER 31
FIRST AID SUPPLIES AND KITS

Once a true regional or national emergency is in progress it will be too late to stock up on medical supplies. Anticipation of a disaster will result in panic buying of medications and sanitary supplies. General civil disorder and looting would certainly result in the loss or destruction of first aid supplies and medications from pharmacies and clinics. Furthermore, hospitals and emergency medical services can be overwhelmed and unavailable in a mass-casualty or epidemic event. Venturing out in search of such supplies under emergency conditions will involve significant risk. The prepared first aider should acquire as much first aid supplies, medical gear, and medications as possible well in advance. These provisions can become critical in rendering care to family members, neighbors, and friends. By being first aid prepared and educated, the first aider is performing an important service to the community. Throughout this book I have identified the specific items needed for various medical emergencies, so this chapter will be devoted to recommendations and lists for kits and packs.

Home First Aid Supplies

First and foremost, stock up on your prescription medications. Acquire any antibiotics and painkillers while you can. Although most medications expire in two years, they are often effective for much longer, especially if vacuum packed and kept cool. You must have a basic first aid book to assure proper procedures. The following is a partial list that could be expanded depending on your needs and skills.

1. 1 pkg., blood stoppers (e.g., Celox™, QuikClot™, HemCon™) powder or dressing
2. 1 (8-oz.) tube, antibiotic ointment (e.g., Neosporin)
3. 1 (8-oz.) tube, hydrocortisone cream

4. 1 (8-oz.) tube burn ointment
5. 1 bar antibacterial soap
6. 12 alcohol swabs
7. 2–4 instant cold packs
8. 1 bottle non-prescription pain medication (e.g., Tylenol™)
9. 1 bottle non-prescription antacid
10. 1 bottle non-prescription antidiuretic
11. 1 bottle non-prescription laxative
12. 1 bottle non-prescription cold and allergy medications
13. 1 (3-oz.) eye drops
14. 1 (2-inch) elastic bandage
15. 1 (3-inch) elastic bandage
16. 2 triangle (cravat) bandages/slings
17. 24 assorted small bandages (e.g., Band-Aid™)
18. 12 (2-inch-square) gauze pads
19. 12 (3-inch-square) gauze pads
20. 12 (4-inch-square) gauze pads
21. 1 (12 inch by 30 inch) multi-trauma dressing
22. 12 safety pins (large)
23. 1 pair EMT shears
24. 1 pair splinter forceps and/or tweezers
25. 4 single-edge razor blades or scalpel blades with blade holder
26. 1 toothache kit (available at drug stores)

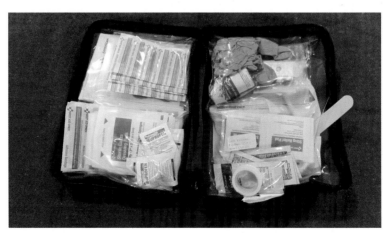

This basic first aid kit from Survival Supply costs about $30 and is adequate for dealing with most minor injuries. It may not be enough to treat more serious injuries and trauma during a disaster survival situation.

27. 6 pair latex gloves your size
28. 1 roll 1-inch self-adhesive tape
29. 1 roll 2-inch self-adhesive tape
30. 1 roll ½-inch medical tape

Other recommended supplies would include a blood pressure cuff and stethoscope to assess a patient's circulatory and respiratory status. Padded aluminum Sam Splints™ are versatile and easy splints that save time. A set of oral airways can be used to prevent the tongue from interfering with a clear airway. While the cervical spine can be stabilized with towels, newspaper and other items, a purpose-made cervical collar is the best method to prevent spinal injury after severe trauma.

Backpack First Aid Kits

Outdoor activities usually involve the risk of some injury. The exact composition of an outdoor first aid kit depends on the potential injuries involved (e.g., hiking vs. rock climbing) and the availability of medical facilities (e.g., local woods vs. deep wilderness). Basic, commercially available first aid kits are usually adequate for day trips or camping in state parks, but more advanced kits or trauma kits may be advisable for those engaging in high-risk activities, and those who venture well beyond the reach of rescue and emergency medical services. The items below would be considered the minimum provisions.

1. Assorted bandages (Band-Aids)
2. Blood stopper (various brands)
3. 4 (3-inch-square) gauze pads
4. Eyewash (1.2 oz.)
5. Single-edge razor blade
6. Splinter tweezers
7. Small scissors
8. Neosporin or triple antibiotic cream
9. Hydrocortisone cream
10. Antacid tablets
11. Laxative tablets
12. Non-prescription pain medication (e.g., ibuprofen, acetaminophen)
13. 2 pairs latex gloves
14. 1-roll self-adhesive tape
15. 1 tourniquet device (e.g., CAT Tourniquet, Israeli Wound Dressing)

Survival Advanced Medical Care Equipment

Beyond basic first aid kits, there are specialized items that can be used by trained individuals to deal with a variety of serious medical emergencies. Advanced medical and surgical supplies were generally unavailable to non-professionals until the development of the internet. Today these items are available to all, and instructions and classes are available online and in various traditional classes specifically for the laymen. Typical advanced medical items include chest seals for closing sucking chest wounds, needle decompression kits for relieving tension pneumothorax and hemothorax, IV setup kits, airway adjuncts, and suturing kits. The HyFin™ vented chest seal, twin packs sell for about $15. TPAK™ needle decompression kits sell for around $10. Nitro-Pak sells basic suturing kits and full emergency surgical kits. They also have larger trauma packs, skin staplers, and airway adjuncts.

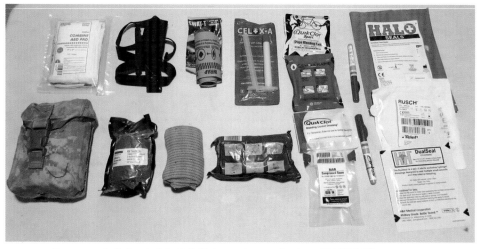

Top row, left to right: CAT™ tourniquet device, SWAT-T™ tourniquet, Celox-A™ hemostatic injector, Quik-Clot™ and Celox hemostatic dressings, ARS™ chest decompression needle kit, HALO™ chest puncture seal. Bottom row, left to right: sterile wound dressing, Israeli combat wound dressing, US military combat wound dressing, small hemostatic dressings, ARS™ chest decompression needle kit, Rusch™ and HH DualSeal™ chest puncture seals.

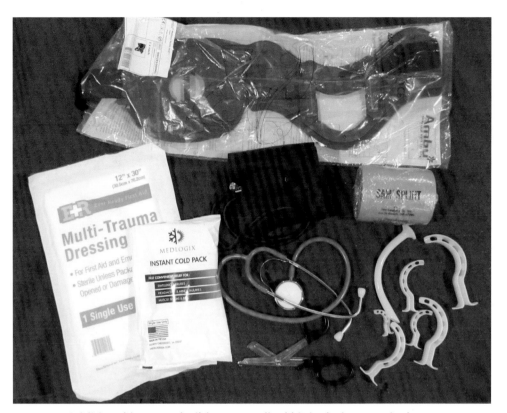

Additional items to build up a medical kit include a cervical collar (top), blood pressure cuff and stethoscope (center), nasal and oral airways (lower right), a Sam Splint™ and large multi-trauma dressings. The EMT shears (bottom center) are excellent for cutting clothing, seatbelts, and bandaging.

Antibiotics

Antibiotics for humans are available only by prescription, but antibiotics for animals can be purchased at farm-supply stores right off the shelf. Fish antibiotics such as cephalexin, doxycycline, and amoxicillin are sold at pet supply stores and through survival supply outlets. BUDK sells a bottle of one-hundred, 250 milligram cephalexin tablets for about $40, the same size amoxicillin goes for $25, and doxycycline at just under $60.

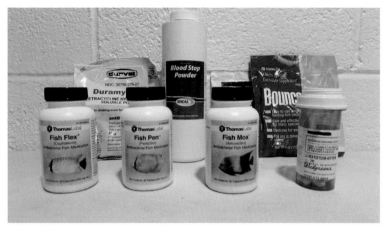

Antibiotics, blood stopper, hydration mix, and other medication can be obtained from veterinary supply and survival supply outlets. While it is generally unwise to retain unused prescription medications, pain medications may be in short supply during a large-scale disaster. Most medications are effective long past the "official" expiration dates.

Surplus Medical Supplies

Flea markets, gun shows, and military surplus outlets often have a variety of high-quality medical supplies and instruments on sale. Out-of-date or obsolete bandaging and dressings are still usable if they remain sealed. Whole combat trauma kits and surgical kits are

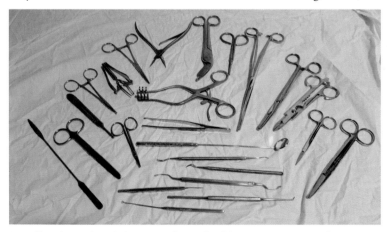

A collection of stainless steel medical instruments purchased at gun shows and flea markets for about one dollar each.

often available. Occasionally, hard to find items such as stretchers and water purifiers can be found. Medical instruments such as clamps, long tweezers, scalpels, scissors, bullet probes, and all sizes of hemostats can be had for a few dollars each. Many medical facilities throw out these expensive tools rather than sterilize them, so they wind up at flea markets or gun shows.

Prepackaged First Aid Kits

If your main concern is just household injuries, then a good basic first aid kit can be purchased online or at local pharmacies, but you may need to supplement it with larger bandages, some two-inch elastic bandages, hemostatic dressings, and various medications for pain and digestive issues.

Trauma Kits

Trauma kits are intended to provide all of the necessary medical equipment to treat and stabilize victims of major injuries, such as arterial bleeding, amputations, sucking chest wounds, large-area burns, and gunshot wounds. Very small kits are designed to be

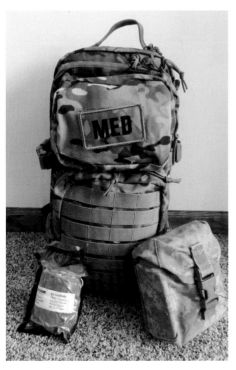

The small Patrol Officers trauma kit on the left from Rescue Essentials™ fits into the pockets of tactical pants and contains a SWAT-T tourniquet gauze and tape. The larger military trauma kit contains a Combat Application Tourniquet (CAT), a wound dressing, and other supplies. The large "Elite Tactical Trauma First Aid Backpack" from Live Action Safety in the center sells for $170 and includes a full cervical collar, tourniquet, major trauma dressings, bandaging, airways, thermal blankets, cold-packs, and other advanced supplies.

carried by police officers and military personnel and are equipped to quickly stop severe bleeding and provide basic wound management pending the arrival at the emergency room or aid station. Larger trauma kits are intended to be carried and used by trained EMT or combat medics, and include more extensive supplies such as cervical collars, wound closure devices, large wound dressings, tape, airways, BP cuffs, stethoscopes, cold packs, Sam Splints™, instruments, and basic personal protective equipment. These larger kits can cost from $130 to over $400 depending on how many victims they are intended to manage.

Should I Invest in an AED?

Automatic Electronic Defibrillation (AED) devices cost thousands of dollars and were only available to professional medics when they first came on the market. These devices have been greatly simplified in recent years so that anyone (I mean anyone) can use them. Lower prices have made them available to install at gyms, schools, and public buildings, but still a bit costly for most home budgets. Lower-cost AEDs have come onto the market very recently and costs may continue to decline. If your household has elderly residents, or those with a high risk for heart attack, investment in an AED may be justified. There is no question that immediate access to and use of an AED by family members can save a life much better than CPR alone.

CHAPTER 32
FIRST AID SKILL TRAINING

There is no substitute for hands-on training in first aid skills. While reading a book about what to do is better than nothing, having to open the book and try a skill for the first time when someone badly needs care is no substitute for just knowing what to do because you have practiced. First aid classes were part of most school curriculum in the past, and the Red Cross offered frequent Basic First Aid and Advanced First Aid course in most communities. The introduction of so-called urgent care facilities in most communities has engendered a culture of dependency and complacency about medical care. The average citizen of today will go to a local urgent care clinic or ER for injuries that were routinely managed at home just a few decades ago.

Recent pandemics and outbreak of civil disorder demonstrated that dependency on system provide medical care is a perilous course. The truly prepared and responsible citizen should be as medically self-sufficient as possible. First aid preparedness is built on four elements.

1. Have at least a few good, well-illustrated first aid manuals that you have actually read and are at least familiar with the content.

2. Have a fully stocked first aid kit including necessary items for wound care, splinting, and primary management of medical conditions without outside support

3. Get training, self-practice, or group practice of basic first aid skills.

4. Continue to acquire and practice more advanced skills and equipment while periodically refreshing basic patient evaluation, triage, and care skills.

Family and Group Self Training

While you may read about how to do a skill, or how to recognize the signs and symptoms of an illness, there is no way to be sure you will do it right without practicing and testing yourself. Buy some bandaging or even tear up some old sheets to make bandages and cravats to practice bandaging and splinting. Have one person pretend to have the symptoms of a condition and let others figure out what the ailment is and what action to take. Go through the motions of airway clearing, CPR, and patient evaluation questions and examination. Try the various rescue techniques while taking care not to injure each other. Learn to work as a team.

For example: One person stabilizes the cervical spine, while another conducts the survey and renders care, and another can get medical supplies. You may even want to set up drill scenarios where one or two members pretend to have injuries or medical emergencies and others have to perform triage and appropriately prioritized care. Another method is to create index cards with the signs and symptoms of an injury or illness. One person can describe or act out the signs and symptoms, and the other members can either verbalize or act out the appropriate (tourniquet, splinting, bandaging, etc.) actions.

Local Survival Prepper Group Classes

Well-organized preparedness organizations can and should conduct first aid training for all members. Community-oriented preparedness groups may want to consider sponsoring open, public first aid classes. The author has developed and conducted numerous training programs, and disaster drills for Live Free USA. I created the Survival Medics course that includes all first aid skills, including suturing, IV setup, and other "beyond first aid" techniques. The course consisted of 8 hours of lecture and Power Point and 8 hours of hands-on practice. I have made the class material (Power Point DVD, outline, handouts, test, etc.), available to anyone with medical qualifications to teach it. Access to CPR mannequins and suture kits are necessary. I also do a three-hour, Eight Critical Medical Skill class that covers airway clearing, CPR, AED, arterial bleeding, hypothermia, hyperthermia, sucking chest wounds, and severe dehydration. I will gladly share these outlines with responsible groups. Preparedness groups can invite paid guest instructors or designate one member to be the group's first aid trainer who can attend advanced classes and then train other members.

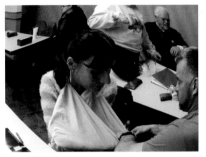

Preparedness groups can conduct first aid training such as this "Survival Medics" class that was open to the public.

Larger groups can conduct realistic disaster drills. A wound simulation kit includes realistic replicas of various wounds including open fractures, amputations, and avulsed intestines.

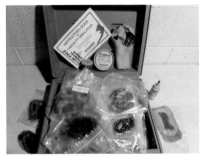

Wound simulation kits are expensive but give a group the ability to conduct realistic training.

The Apprentice Doctor Kits

Some of the best self-training systems available to the public are sold by The Apprentice Doctor at www.theapprenticedoctor.com. Their kits include everything the student needs to learn and practice basic and advanced medical skills. The Future Doctors kit contains a training course and all the simulations to practice basic examination and patient evaluation skills, priced at $99. The IV Phlebotomy kit includes all of the material to learn how to set up an intravenous line, including syringes, needles, tubing, and a simulated arm to practice IV setup for $119. Their orthopedic fractures reduction training kit sells for under $200. A Control Bleeding training kit includes a simulated arterial bleed and a tourniquet device. The Apprentice Doctor's suturing training kit and course sells for $79.

Using these kits, an individual, family, or group can acquire advanced medical skills not generally available to the public.

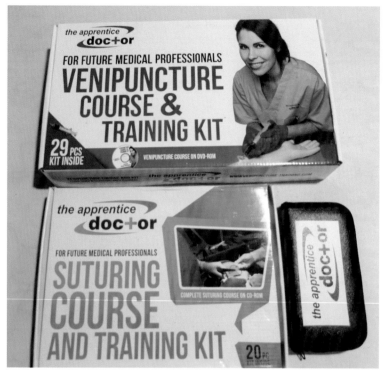

The Apprentice Doctor training kits include everything you need to master a variety of advanced medical skills.

First Aid Certifications

While certification is a desirable goal, and necessary for employment in some professions, it is not essential for the citizen first aider who renders emergency care. The possession of a certificate does not affect your coverage under the Good Samaritan Laws in any way. If you know the skill, and do your best, that's all that counts. No one's life was ever saved by a piece of paper or lack thereof. I have encountered people who were afraid to do CPR because their certification had expired. I know people that will not use an AED because they are not certified. While certification courses are usually well-done and well-intended, they often engender the idea that certification is necessary to perform the procedure and action without an up-to-date certificate is illegal. This is not the case.

CPR/AED Classes

Cardiopulmonary Resuscitation and Automatic Electronic Defibrillator training classes are available online through the American Red Cross,

American Heart Association, National Safety Council, and other agencies, at a wide range of prices. Hands-on and combination hands-on and online classes are also available, and locations and schedules can be found on their websites. Schools, churches, community organizations and local health care agencies also may sponsor CPR/AED courses.

Become a First Responder

First responder courses provide an opportunity to attain a nationally recognized medical care certification. These courses include CPR, AED, control of severe bleeding, and most basic first aid skills. While online courses are available, hands-on programs may be found through your local fire department. Your employer may even sponsor OSHA first responder courses. First responder certification requires 50 hours of training and the student must pass a written and scenario-based practical test.

Become an EMT

Emergency medical technician courses are usually enrolled in by those seeking employment at a fire department, ambulance service, or medical facility. Certification as an EMT, B (Basic) requires 120 hours of training, passing a 60- to 100-question written examination, and a set of scenario-based hands-on tests. EMT programs are managed through state departments of Homeland Security (DHS) and local courses can be found through that agency. These courses cost from 800 to 1,000 dollars, but the cost may be paid by the local fire department or employing sponsor. Being a National Registered EMT qualifies the recipient to apply for employment in an ambulance or medical care facility, and it is the first step to becoming an EMT-A (advanced) or an EMT-P (paramedic). These advanced training levels are only available through sponsoring agencies.

Become a Certified Nurse's Assistant (CNA)

Under emergency conditions the health care system may be overwhelmed or even collapse, leaving citizens to provide long-term care for family members. CNA courses are not oriented towards first aid but focus on basic patient care, such as movement and handling of the disabled, recognition of developing health issues, dietary management, bathing, and monitoring of vital signs. CNAs usually work under the supervision of a nurse or doctor, but if you have elderly family members, or someone you know is experiencing a prolonged recovery, becoming a CNA may be of value. Licensed and certified CNAs are in demand for jobs at nursing homes and hospitals. You may even be eligible to become a paid caregiver for a family member. Training is often available at community colleges for $400 to $1,000, but employers may pay part or all of the cost.

Volunteer for Community Service

Preparedness is responsible citizenship. The best way to keep your family safe is to help keep your community safe, by being part of the community's disaster response and public safety programs. Participation in these programs provides training and puts you in a better position to anticipate and survive crime, civil disorder, epidemics, and other hazardous situations. After the events of September 11, 2001, the federal government initiated several programs intended to support citizen involvement in disaster response. Two of the most successful are the Civilian Emergency Response Teams (CERTS) and the Volunteers in Police Services (VIPS) programs.

CIVILIAN EMERGENCY RESPONSE TEAMS (CERTs)

Some CERTs groups are fairly small and underfunded while others have scores of members and their own vehicles and trailers. The initial CERTs curriculum of training includes emergency preparedness, basic first aid, light search and rescue, and fire extinguisher training. The training culminates in a short disaster drill with simulated entrapped and injured victims. In the event of an emergency, their tasks would include house-to-house checks for victims and marking the house as checked. Of course, if injured living occupants are found they can provide basic extrication and first aid and use their radios to call for further assistance. Wrenches are carried to turn off the gas valves to damaged structures. Doing these basic tasks relieves the fire, police, and EMS to focus on the more serious situations.

CERTs members are issued a backpack containing a flashlight, water containers, heavy-gloves, safety goggles, a hard-hat, knee-pads, crowbar, first aid kit, glow-sticks, and various other supplies. They also get a visibility vest, cap, and photo identification card. CERTs groups are usually organized by the local fire department, and instructors must attend a certified trainer's course. Periodic review meetings are required. If your town or county has a CERTs program you should give it your full support and participation. If not,

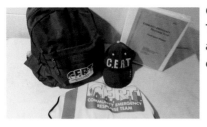

Civilian Emergency Response Teams are trained in first aid and rescue skills and issued equipment and identification.

encourage your town to establish a CERTs program. For information go to: www.ready.gov/cert

VOLUNTEERS IN POLICE SERVICE (VIPS)

These programs may exist under various titles (police auxiliaries, police reserves, etc.) and be accomplished in a variety of ways, but the VIPS program was initiated after 9/11 and follows guidelines supported by the International Association of Chiefs of Police. Some towns combine the disaster response responsibilities of CERTs and the police support activities into one organization. VIPS (by whatever name) members are not armed and are not assigned to hazardous duties. They may patrol on foot, bicycle, or vehicle to observe and report. Vehicular patrols perform such duties as crime scene protection, parking enforcement, checking houses where owners are on vacation, and opened and closed business checks. VIPS volunteers may also be assigned traffic control duties or pedestrian control duties at special events or may use their vehicles to escort funerals or protect disabled vehicles waiting to be towed. In an emergency situation, they can also be used to help with crowd control. VIPS members also can work at the police station helping with records and other office duties. At no time are they expected to pursue, confront, or arrest anyone.

These programs are generally under the police or public safety department's management. The extent of training will depend on the organizers and the local leadership. Candidates are screened carefully and put through extensive training as if they are actual police officers. After an interview with police officials, candidates' records are run through the federal and state databases, put through an extensive psychological evaluation, and then a basic physical.

Training subjects include the following: police procedures, confidentiality, records and documentation, first aid, CPR/AED, blood borne pathogens, radio protocols, patrolling techniques, fingerprinting, use of the Spillman™ computer system, and driving the special

VIPS police vehicle. One thing that is emphasized strongly is that we do not talk to anyone (I mean anyone) about anything we see or hear related to the police department, crimes, or anything else. Since VIPS do not carry weapons (and are prohibited from carrying), they do not usually get firearms training. VIPS are issued a modified uniform, jacket, radio, flashlight, gear belt, and in some cases full bulletproof vest. A minimum number of service hours is usually required. While VIPS are not cops they are respected by the police officers as (in their words) the "ultimate examples of responsible citizens." VIPS and similar programs require a serious commitment from the participant. This is not playing police. This is taking a highly responsible, part-time job without pay, but it can certainly be an educational and gratifying experience that helps to protect you, your family, and your community. For further information go to www.theiacp.org/VIPS

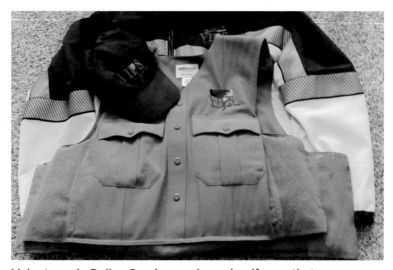

Volunteers in Police Service are issued uniforms that may even include a bulletproof vest. They carry radios and drive police-like vehicles but are not armed.

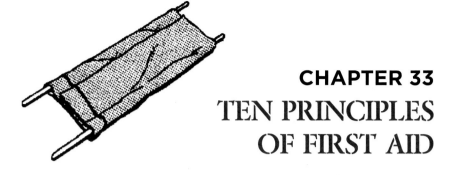

CHAPTER 33
TEN PRINCIPLES
OF FIRST AID

These principles are derived from my "Ten Principles of Survival" and provide a fitting conclusion to this book. These principles apply to virtually any situation; in fact, they apply to life in general. In analyzing disaster responses, business activities, industrial accidents, and individual life situations, I have found that when these principles were applied, successful outcomes or at least the best possible outcomes were achieved, whereas failures and disasters could always be traced to failure to apply one or more of these principles. The ten principles apply especially well to rendering first aid under emergency conditions and are integral to elements of the chapters of this book.

1. Anticipate

On a primary level, anticipation of the need to be able to render first aid in an emergency has driven your quest for knowledge and skill. Anticipation has opened your mind to the potential of injury and illness when you may be the first responder or even the only responder. You are taking responsibility in anticipation of the need by learning skills and acquiring equipment. Your life or the life of others may be saved because you anticipated the possibility, prepared, and were able to act. What kinds of medical emergencies you anticipate depends on your age, location, health, and life situation. Unfortunately, natural disasters, civil unrest, violent crime, and terrorism must be added to home accidents and normal illnesses as sources of medical emergencies we can anticipate.

On a more immediate level, the first aider must know how to anticipate the kinds of developments that a given type of injury or illness will create. You will need to anticipate the development of shock in a patient who has lost a lot of blood. You need to anticipate a declining level of consciousness for a head injury patient. In many cases you will need to anticipate a heart attack or other serious development before it occurs and initiate transportation to professional care. You can anticipate the development of hypothermia or hyperthermia from early signs and symptoms and prevent the development of these life-threatening conditions.

2. Be Aware

Scene safety is the first step in responding to any emergency. Awareness of the environment and dangers are essential to keeping you from becoming just another victim. Confined spaces may hold toxic gases or be oxygen deficient. Street situations may involve armed criminals. A "bystander" may in fact be the assailant. In a natural disaster or accident, downed electric lines, leaking flammables, and unstable structures or vehicles may pose a hazard to the responder. Being aware of the hazards posed by communicable diseases and hazardous chemicals is critical to assuring that you wear the proper respiratory, eye, and skin protection.

Being aware requires that you avoid "tunnel vision" on the first or most spectacular victim you encounter. A screaming, thrashing victim has an airway and a high level of consciousness, whereas a silent victim behind that door you came in or on the other side of the vehicle may need immediate action to restore breathing or stop severe bleeding.

3. Be Here Now

This principle always sounds a bit strange, but it can be very important. Under the pressure of a medical emergency the "fight or flight" instinct may push you, or at least your mind, to be somewhere else. You may start thinking about how to pass this on to others, or just walk away. Maybe no one knows that you know first aid, but you know. Maybe instead of running to help you pretend you didn't know what happened. Maybe you start worrying more about what will happen if you make a mistake than what will happen if you do nothing. Facing a serious medical emergency on your own can be a very stressful time, but you must act. Even if your mind goes blank (this is normal), once you start doing your scene safety, PPE, and patient evaluation it will come back to you, if you have studied and trained. As a trainer myself, I know people who flunked every written test but once thrown into a simulated practical scenario performed every skill perfectly. Get your head into the moment.

4. Stay Calm

Easy to say on paper but hard to do in practice. Experienced EMTs do become able to handle mass casualties, blood, screaming, and making life and death decisions calmly, but the citizen first aider who has seldom if ever faced such circumstances is going to be nervous. The body's normal reaction will pump adrenaline into to the system, increase respirations and heart rate, and cause mental paralysis and tunnel vision. Training and anticipation can overcome some of this. If you seem to be calm, then everyone else, including the patient or patients, will be calmer. Telling a patient that is obviously about to have a heart attack that "It's probably nothing, but let's check things out," may postpone the actual attack. Pretending to be calm is actually a critical first aid skill that comforts the patient and actually helps to calm the first aider. Comments like "This is very, very bad," or "Oh my god!" will not help anyone.

5. Evaluate

This goes directly to chapters 5 and 7 that cover triage and patient evaluation. You can't treat it properly if you don't accurately identify the problem. Being able to quickly identify the need for immediate lifesaving action and then move on to identify and treat other injuries and illness on conscious and unconscious patients is an important first aid skill. These are basic EMT skills but often ignored in "first aid" books. These books assume that the injury or illness will be obvious (e.g., broken leg, cardiac arrest), but patient evaluation skills are critical to identification of primary and secondary medical issues when professional medical support is not available. In fact, evaluation of the injury and illness in relation to the availability of professional medical help is important to decision making. Should you try to reset a dislocation, or remove a bullet, if support will be long delayed? Should you move or remove a patient from a vehicle or building, or wait for help? Evaluation of potential risk versus potential benefits of your actions is an ongoing process.

6. Do the Next Right Thing

This is the essence of the Hippocratic Oath: "Do no further harm." The next right thing may be CPR or application of a tourniquet. Often calling 911 is the first right thing. The sequence of right things is usually scene safety, triage (if needed), securing an airway, restoring breathing and circulation, stopping severe bleeding, treating for shock, and then bandaging, splinting, and other first aid as needed. In some cases, simply calming the patient and doing your patient evaluation is the next right thing. Moving a severely injured victim with potential spinal injuries when they are in a safe place and help is on the way would not be the "right thing," but doing so using the techniques in this book when the victim is in danger and no help is anticipated may be "the next right thing." While doing nothing is seldom the "right thing," making reckless decisions that endanger the patient without justification is never "the next right thing." Think before you act.

7. Take Control

Like it or not, you are in charge once you initiate first aid. Give orders! Send others for help. Have others bring first aid gear, blankets, AEDs, etc. Show others how to do CPR when you are exhausted. Have others or even the patient hold dressings in place or help with splint application. If others claim to know first aid skills or CPR, let them help under your supervision, but you cannot step away from the patient unless and until professional emergency responders arrive or you have handed off the patient at the hospital. Bystanders and family members are inclined to criticize and question your actions, but do not let them distract you from doing the right thing. If you can assign someone to keep bystanders away, do so. Patient privacy is important. You can calmly explain what you are doing and why, but don't be told what to do or not to do by panicked and untrained bystanders. Putting others to work keeps them out of your way. When treating multiple victims, you can ask less injured to help you with the severely injured first, this keeps them occupied and calm until you can attend to them. You are in charge, or chaos will reign.

8. Have What You Need

The old adage, "Better to have it and not need it, than need it and not have it," applies double to medical emergencies. Having the skills and equipment you need when you need it and where you need it can mean life and or death to someone you care about. Chapters 31 and 32 cover various ways to acquire more first aid skills and an extensive selection of first aid kits and advanced trauma care equipment. One of my mantras is, "It's not what you have, but what you have with you that counts." Having well-selected first aid kits in your vehicle and pack is a must, but having a few first aid items as "everyday carry" in your pocket or purse is also essential. A compact tourniquet or at least a bandana that can be used as an improvised tourniquet or bandage should always be handy. An N95 dust mist respirator can provide protection from biological, chemical, and particulate hazards in a disaster. Even a few Band-Aids and gauze pads can come in handy. If you are on prescription medications, don't assume you can get home; have a few days' supply with you. At home you can and should have a complete supply of first aid equipment, first aid books, and sanitation supplies for a long-lasting disaster situation. The pandemic of 2020 certainly demonstrated that hospitals and clinics can be overwhelmed or dangerous places to be avoided if possible. Things like oxygen, AEDs, surgical instruments, antibiotics, and advanced pain medications may be needed in the gravest extremes.

9. Use What You Have

The ability to improvise is an essential survival skill, and even more so in first aid situations. No matter how well you plan and equip, you may not have the ideal item to manage a medical emergency. The bare hand or any piece of cloth can be used to apply direct pressure to a wound. A bandana or belt can be used as a tourniquet. Newspaper or cardboard can serve as an improvised splint. A blanket, a board, or even a door can be used as a litter to move a patient. Rolled-up towels can form a cervical spine splint. Plastic wrap can be used to cover a wound or secure a splint. Duct tape or electrical tape can secure a dressing or splint. It doesn't have to be pretty; it just has to work.

10. Do What Is Necessary

This is an essential principle because responding to medical emergencies under survival conditions can involve some unpleasant situations and hard decisions. For starters, you may find yourself working in blood, vomit, urine, and other unpleasant substances. EMTs carry mouth wash in their kits because patients often vomit, causing the EMT to vomit as well. You may have to be firm with patients and bystanders in order to perform the necessary procedures. While patient comfort is desirable, splinting, bandaging, and other actions may cause them some pain and complaints. Do what you must do. In multiple injury scenarios, you may need to ignore a non-critical, screaming patient or even a child in order to perform lifesaving action on another patient. In the gravest extreme you may be required triage patients, and even decide that one or more patients cannot be saved and move on to critical but salvageable patients. Do what you have to do.

11. Never Give Up

In addition to the ten principles, there always has to be one over-reaching rule. While triage may determine that you prioritize care to the most salvageable patients, most cases will involve only a few patients and permit some level of comfort care for even the most severely injured and terminal patients. Obviously massive and multiple injuries to the head or torso are seldom survivable, but the human body is capable of amazing things. In the 1800s, a trapper had his gut torn open and was left in the woods to die. Many days later he walked into Fort Michilimackinac in Michigan with a healed open stomach. A physician there used him to study how food is digested. A woman in Tennessee rode on horseback to the doctor with a soft-ball-sized tumor in her abdomen. The doctor removed it without anesthetics or antibiotics, and she rode home on a horse and lived a long life. People have recovered from severe hypothermia, engendering the medical paradigm that "no one is dead until they are warm dead." A girl in Pakistan was shot in the head at close range with an AK-47 and lived to address the UN. Do your best. Do what you can for everyone. Have faith and hope for the best.

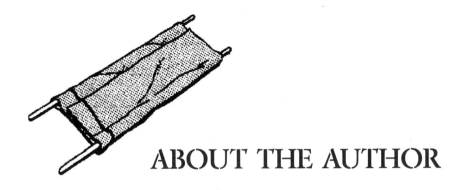

ABOUT THE AUTHOR

James C. Jones was born on the Southside of Chicago at the beginning of World War II. An impoverished and chaotic childhood made him a natural survivalist from a very early age. He put together his own survival pack at age twelve and often spent time in the woodlands and swamps that adjoined the city at that time. Working two jobs while living in one room and attending high school in the tough Southside added more real-world survival experiences. Starting as a technician at a large chemical manufacturing complex, his passion for safety led him to become an award-winning safety manager. While acquiring certifications as an emergency medical technician (EMT), Hazardous Material Technician, Hazard Control Manager, Safety Manager, and Training Manager, he energetically pursued survival-related activities including rock climbing, caving, white water rafting, horseback riding, and survival camping. His training allowed him to combine safety science, human behavior, and personal experience in developing programs and publications directed at helping responsible citizens become more self-reliant and better prepared to survive emergencies. He founded Live Free USA in the late 1960s and helped it evolve from an outdoor survival club into a broad-based, national preparedness and self-reliance education organization. During the 1970s and 1980s, he was a leading voice in defending and defining responsible survivalism on national television and radio and even the BBC.

James C. Jones is the author of four books: *Advanced Survival, Total Survival, 150 Survival Secrets*, and *The Ultimate Guide to Survival Gear*, all published by Skyhorse Publishing. He has developed and conducted hundreds of survival training events and seminars over the past forty years. Now retired and living in Indiana, he currently writes articles for several national preparedness and survival related publications, including Live Free USA's "American Survivor" newsletter and website at www.americansurvivor.org, while continuing to teach a variety of survival courses and make presentations at major preparedness expositions.